Praise for Choco.... Yoga

"As a women's health educator and coach I have been practicing yoga since I was a young girl and I am always seeking new ways to educate women to the value of a daily practice of yoga. **Chocolate Yoga** has beautifully captured the essence of yoga while inviting the reader to embark on the journey through a simple and joyful approach. Author Margaret Chester embraces the "art of living" by providing tools for dealing with the challenges of life. Her words are uplifting and a sweet companion to every day. If you have never done yoga this is a great book to get you on the path and if you are a life-long student of yoga you will find joy in this new approach."

~ Wendy Mitchell, MA, CPC

"I find my **Chocolate Yoga** several times a day while standing in front of my refrigerator. I no longer bother to open the door. Instead I stand quietly and slowly take five deep breaths. I am then ready to walk away, usually singing or humming, 'I got along without you before I met you, gonna get along without you now.' I feel so victorious. **Chocolate Yoga** is definitely my favorite snack."

~ Shirley B.

"This book is a life saver. I started a new job about the time that I started reading **Chocolate Yoga.** The job is stressful to say the least. Taking a moment every couple of hours to stop and breathe and do an internal lift has made all the difference in the world."

~ B.A. Mayler, Bellingham, WA

"I absolutely loved **Chocolate Yoga.** Whenever I'm feeling overloaded with commitments and chores, Margaret Chester's common-sense, yet comforting suggestions bring me instant peace. I can honestly say this book changed my life."

~ Susan Colleen Browne,
author of *Little Farm in the Foothills* and *Little Farm Homegrown*

"While doing the layout and design of this book I found the concepts and suggestions to be invaluable. I used the *Chocolate Yoga* breathing techniques to stay calm during biopsies and surgery. I'm sure this book helped me with my swift recovery."

~ Kate Weisel, Bellingham, WA

"This slim tome is filled with inspiring passages and techniques of how we can withhold snippets of our own days—just for ourselves. Margaret names these blessed moments "chocolate." She uses chocolate as a metaphor for those moments in time that nourish the soul. A few moments here, a few moments there when we are mindful of our breathing will make a difference. Exhale. Inhale. Breathe. These few moments a day of me nurturing me was making a difference."

~ Chanticleer Book Reviews & Media

"*Chocolate Yoga* is filled with inspiring passages and techniques, trail-blazing an entirely different approach to stress and weight management. It describes a way of life, brought to us in a reader-friendly, body-friendly guide to the basics of yoga. Not just mechanical poses or asanas, but a more mindful, well-rounded approach to health and life."

~ Matt McErlean

Yoga for Ageless Seniors

Daily Prescriptions for Increasing Strength, Balance & Resilience

Margaret Chester, MPH, RYT

Yoga for Ageless Seniors:
Daily Prescriptions for Increasing Strength, Balance & Resilience

Copyright © 2019 by Margaret Chester

All right reserved

(www.chocolateyoga.com)

First edition, 2019

ISBN: 978-0-9831882-4-7 (paperback)
ISBN: 978-0-9831882-5-4 (e-book)

Book design and typography, plus e-book preparation
by Kathleen R. Weisel (www.weiselcreative.com)

Dedication

To all the elders in my life,
who have given me the courage to carry on
despite the never-ending roadblocks,
adversity, heartaches, and pain.
This is my thank you to all of you.

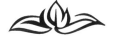

A Brief Note Before We Begin

This is not a technical, scientific, or scholarly treatise. It is my interpretation of applying the principles of yoga to the aging process. Please consult a licensed health care practitioner for professional medical advice before making any changes in your routine. This includes seeking financial, legal, and real estate advice from a licensed professional.

Disclaimers

This publication contains the opinions and ideas of its author. It provides helpful and informative material on the subject matter covered. It is sold with the understanding that the author and publisher are not engaged in rendering professional services in the book. If the reader requires personal assistance or advice, a competent professional should be consulted.

The author and publisher specifically disclaim any responsibility for any liability, loss, injury or damage, personal or otherwise, incurred as a consequence, directly or indirectly, of the use and application of any of the information contained in this book.

If you have any major health issues, please consult a licensed health care practitioner before you begin this program. You are responsible for setting limits for yourself at all times.

This is NOT a proven medical science program. The author is not a licensed healthcare professional. It is an experiential system that may or may not work for you. The author is offering you ideas that will help you connect with your true self.

Under no circumstances should you ignore any symptoms that may require a diagnosis, treatment, and active care by a licensed health care practitioner.

This yoga is not intended to diagnose, treat, cure, or prevent any condition or disease.

Thank you Frances for your editing tenacity,
and Kate for your incredible patience
in design and typography.
All mistakes are mine.

Contents

Welcome to
Yoga for Ageless Seniors

Growing older is the most fascinating and repulsive pro-cess that I have ever encountered in my sixty-five plus years. My chronologically older friends and relatives have told me: *Just you wait, you haven't seen anything yet.* For years I have read everything I could on aging, dying, and death. I was sincerely hoping to figure out how to skip the wrinkles, age spots, sagging skin, memory loss, insomnia, muscle decline, an urge to nap after every meal along with urinary inconti-nence, failing eyesight, spontaneous farts, and an expanding middle.

It is not just the reality of taking care of my aging physi-cal body that concerns me, but the reality that anything can happen to me or my loved ones at any time. Every day I hear a horror story along the lines of: *I just went into the kitchen to make a cup of tea and the next thing I knew, I was on the floor in pain. After the emergency room, an MRI, hip surgery and six weeks in a rehab center, I will never get back into shape.* The truth is that we do not bounce back from physical trau-mas as quickly as when we were sixteen years old.

And then there is that long list of possible diagnoses, in-cluding but not limited to: *accidents, ALS, Alzheimer's, de-mentia, cancer, diabetes, heart disease, kidney disease, multi-ple sclerosis, Parkinson's, respiratory diseases, strokes, sudden falls, suicide, and long-term care.* If I do get a diagnosis and treatment or face some mysterious unidentifiable illness – how will I deal with the stress? How can I learn to deal with the known and the unknown – including my guaranteed dying and death? Is there any way to build up my resilience to the above which includes living fully until I die?

I wanted a checklist, a guide, a sage, a mentor to nudge me into paying attention to living my life as fully as I can – until I die. Based on my readings and experiences, I decided to write my own prescriptions, using the five ancient yoga techniques outlined in *Chocolate Yoga for Stress and Weight Management* and *The Chocolate Yoga Workbook*.

Please take all my ideas with a grain of salt, sugar or honey! These yoga techniques have been around for ages and this is just my spin on them. And yes, I am aware that some chapters are shorter than others, that my yoga ideas will upset some people, and that the Appendix could stand alone as a workbook or a workshop. I wrote this book for me, and if it can assist just one person live a fuller, juicier, more audacious life – then I am pleased to have been a contributor.

We are the wise seniors and the sage elders of the land so it is our responsibility to set a good example on how to live fully until we die. May *Yoga for Ageless Seniors* assist you in adding more pleasure, mindfulness, and smiles to the last few chapters of your life. May it also give you the courage to carry *OM* – no matter what may come your way.

Namaste,
Margaret Chester
2019

Food for Thought

"On my last birthday, I was ninety-three years old.

That is not young, of course.

In fact, it is older than ninety.

But age is a relative matter.

If you continue to work and to absorb the beauty

in the world about you –

you find that age does not necessarily mean getting old.

At least, not in the ordinary sense.

I feel many things more intensely than ever before,

and for me, life grows more fascinating."

— Pablo Cassals, *Joys and Sorrows* (1970)

Please Do Not Let
The Word
"YOGA"
Turn You
Off —
If
You
Can
Breathe
You
Can
Do
This
Yoga!

Introduction

*Why bother caring about your body, mind, and spirit
if you are just going to die anyway?*

Yes, you and I are going to die someday. *Why bother doing this yoga? Why even try?* And my answer is: *Why not?* If you could give yourself a few more minutes of pleasure every day without spending a penny – wouldn't you be interested? Here's your reward:

1. **Aging:** Yoga is an *all-in-one* system that will give you increased strength, balance, and resilience in your body, mind, and spirit.

2. **Stress management:** Yoga reduces the physical effects of stress on the body and the mind – making it easier to handle your personal stress issues.

3. **Pain relief:** Numerous studies have found that a combination of movement, breathing, and meditation can ease physical, emotional, and mental pain.

4. **Improved breathing:** Increased oxygen in the body produces positive brain activity.

5. **Flexibility:** Practicing yoga can increase your range of motion, improve muscle tone, and body alignment.

6. **Increased strength:** Yoga postures will build muscle power and help protect your bones.

7. **Cardiovascular conditioning:** Practicing yoga will improve circulation and lower your resting heart rate. It will also increase your endurance and oxygen intake as you do any movement or exercise.

8. **Inner peace:** The meditative aspects of practicing yoga will give you a lifetime of tools for dealing with reality. This practice will help you make peace with your past, present, and future.

9. **Yoga is FREE:** We are all on a budget and if we pay for something, we want to get our money's worth. The good news is that yoga is FREE and you can access it anytime and anywhere. No gym memberships, special equipment, or expensive clothing are required.

There is no quick fix or magic pill for healing our body, mind, and spirit. We still need to deal with backed-up toilets, traffic jams, snowstorms, cancelled flights, positive biopsies, family rifts, taxes, death, dying, and the endless changes in our internal and external life. The aging process is here to stay, so please take a deep breath and work with what you have today. My goal is to give you some ideas that you will incorporate, modify, and change to fit your everyday needs.

WARNING: We Are Going To Discuss Death And Dying!

The ancient yogis were very much aware that death follows life and that one can practice dying every day with joy, awareness and gratitude. In fact, your life will become lighter and happier once you acknowledge that you will eventually die and that the choices you make today really count with every breath that you take. This entire yoga practice is all about adding more pleasure, mindfulness, and smiles into your everyday life. Feel free to skip to the APPENDIX at any time to check out what I like to call Homework. Remember, if you do not live your life, who will?

Before we go any further,

I would like you to

Gently place your hand between your breasts,

At your heart center

And promise yourself

To love, honor, and cherish

Your body, mind, and spirit.

From this day forward.

My Definitions

The following are my definitions that I will be using throughout *Yoga for Ageless Seniors.*

Yoga is simply: "The cessation of the chattering of the mind," as defined in the *Sutras* of *Patanjali.* In other words, yoga is simply being here right now in this very moment. If you are breathing mindfully – you are *"doing"* yoga. Yoga is most frequently defined as a series of postures, meditations, and breathing exercises. Please note that there are many schools of yoga, philosophies, and systems. *Yoga for Ageless Seniors* is just my spin on an ancient system for creating health, internal wealth, and happiness.

Ageless in *Yoga for Ageless Seniors* simply refers to living your best life today. *Ageless* implies the ability to be in the moment with no beginning and no end. Imagine your thoughts, actions, and deeds as seedlings that you are planting throughout your life, that will continue to grow and blossom long after you are gone.

Seniors refers to anyone who has survived sixty or more years of living life. It also refers to those who manifest wisdom.

Techniques are specialized procedures and methods, used in any field, in which people of all ages and walks of life apply skills to affect a desired result.

Daily refers to something that is done, occurring, or issued every day or night.

Prescriptions are directions traditionally written by a medical practitioner to a pharmacist for the preparation and dosage of a medicine or remedy. I am using the idea of a prescription as a course of action that you self-administer.

Strength is used here as the qualities of being strong in body, mind, and/or spirit.

Balance refers to being in a state of equilibrium, stability, evenness, or steadiness. It also implies the reality of yin/yang and how the body, mind, and spirit are constantly striving to achieve homeostasis.

Resilience is the ability to recover and heal from adversity, illness, depression, grief, or any life-altering event.

On a Daily Basis is an activity that is carried out at least once a day to contribute to the maintenance of the body, mind, and spirit.

Additional Definitions
that I will be using throughout this book are:

Body as in the physical structure of a person.

Mind as in the human part of the body that reasons, thinks, feels, wills, perceives, judges, and makes up stories.

Spirit as in the principle of living a conscious life. It is used in this book interchangeably with the word *breath.*

Please note that I will also be using the word **health** as a person's overall attitude. I am not using it in the usual "free from illness or injury" sense, because I believe that we are more than our diagnosis, wounds, and injuries. The word **health** has roots in the word **whole,** as in "a thing that is complete in itself." Therefore, actions and non-actions that support the whole person in body, mind, spirit, and emotions can result in optimal health and wellness. *Yoga for Ageless Seniors* is simply about creating healthy, happy, and sacred moments every day.

The Five Elements

Daily

Prescriptions

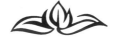

The Five Elements: Mix & Match

1. **Breathing**

2. **Internal Contractions**

3. **Gazing In & Out**

4. **Movement**

5. **Rest & Relaxation**

These techniques may be practiced individually or in any combination. You will notice that I do not say: *hold for two breaths* or *repeat three times.* I leave those details up to you. The variations of these five elements are limitless, so have fun using these ideas and make sure that you tailor each technique to meet your individual needs. These skills are very portable; you may do them anytime and anywhere. You may find yourself drawn to one aspect of the practice for weeks or even months. As with a favorite food, we often crave what we need, what is comfortable, and feels good in the moment! *This is your yoga – do only what works for you today.*

Ground Rules and Guidelines

The best way to practice *Yoga for Ageless Seniors* is to pretend you are at a huge buffet – try anything that looks and sounds good. If you like it, go back for seconds. If you don't like it – let it go.

- Start with the body that you have today. Remember to honor your injuries, surgeries, and physical limitations. This includes muscle/joint issues, chronic illnesses, or ailments.

- Practicing yoga is NOT about creating discomfort or causing harm – it is all about releasing tension.

- Pain is the messenger: Listen to your body and your mind. If you experience any sharp pains, please back off – this also includes emotional pain. I am assuming you are a responsible person, so please assess the situation honestly and seek professional help as needed. Part of staying healthy is knowing when you need assistance and reaching out to find a helping hand.

- Remember, this is not a contest. Have fun. Challenge yourself to lighten up, laugh, and turn the page.

Food for Thought

"My actions are my only true belongings."

— Thích Nhất Hạnh

ELEMENT ONE

The Power of Breathing: Breath is Life

I have been doing yoga for years, but I never really understood the breathing part until I worked in a hospice program. The nurses used the term *Cheyne-Stokes* – a breathing pattern of taking several rapid breaths followed by a period of seemingly not breathing. The first time I witnessed it, it was a bit like sleep apnea. I held my breath waiting for the dying person to take their next breath. I watched as their breaths got further and further apart until there was nothing. No chest rising, no pulse, and no heartbeat. Then I got it. Life is breath, and if you are not breathing, you are dead.

NOTE: *I do know that there are machines that can help you breathe; however, that is a discussion for you to have with your family/friends, physician, and advanced directive team.*

With every death I witnessed, I was totally humbled by the power of the breath. I no longer work in the hospice field, but it helped me to become more attuned to the simple joy of being able to breathe. To this day, I try to check in mindfully with my breath several times a day – simply to thank my heart and lungs for taking care of me.

Definition of Breathe, Breath & Breathing

I will be using *breathe, breath,* and *breathing* as the act of taking oxygen into the lungs and expelling it, as in respiration. *Breathing* also refers to spirit, soul, wind, animation, vigor, and force. The Greek roots *pneuma* (breath) and *psycheim* (to breathe) and the Latin rook *spiritus* (breath) may all be linked to the words we use today: breath, life, psyche, soul, spiritual, and respiratory. The German word *brodem* refers to *vapor,* Old English *broedam* refers to *burn* and Old High German *bradam* to *heat* and *breathe.* Other words that refer to breath and breathing are: *chi* (Chinese), *ha* (Hawaiian), *ki* (Japanese), *mana* (Malayo-Polynesian), *neshamah* (Hebrew) *orenda* (Native American), *ruach* (Hebrew-Aramaic) and *prana* (Sanskrit). In the following prescriptions, you will see how the breath can be used to soothe one's ruffled feathers, pause, and take a much needed break, or stoke the fires and get moving!

Most of us think of breathing as just inhaling and exhaling. But did you know that the **pause** is the most underrated and misunderstood part of the breathing cycle? The pause between the inhaling and exhaling is where the magic happens. Think about it. *I want a cookie.* If I really take a deep breath, pause for a few seconds and then exhale very slowly, I can allow my body/mind to connect and say: *Really, Margaret, you don't want a cookie, you are just delaying that uncomfortable phone call.* Now I have a choice: eat the cookie and delay the phone call, or ignore the cookie and go make that phone call. Or better yet, I often tell myself that I can have a cookie after I make that phone call!

Another example of using the **pause** in real life is when you have to deal with receiving upsetting news: *the car needs a major repair; you need a biopsy; a friend just died; or there has been another random shooting or an airplane crash.* Our knee-jerk reaction is usually to react immediately with anger, disbelief, shock, sadness, or depression. Then we may churn the event over and over to ourselves, or repeat the same story to friends or anyone who will listen. I am not saying that it is wrong to process; however, you may first want to try some deep breathing techniques and see what happens. Really listen to the **pause** between each breath. The pause will give your body and your mind a chance to connect. You may even get an insight of what you can do on a very practical level to deal with *the car, the biopsy, a friend's death, a shooting event* or *a plane crash.* Listen closely to your insights, because they will guide you into living your truth. Remember, breathing is a sacred gift to be treasured from birth to death; honor that gift by breathing fully for the rest of your life.

Yoga Rx:
The Power of Breathing

The following five breathing techniques are offered as suggestions. Please feel free to adjust and personalize each one according to your daily needs.

1. **Three Part Breathing**

2. **The Secret Power of the Pause**

3. **Sealed with a Kiss**

4. **Heart Centered Breathing**

5. **Breathing Meditation**

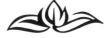

1. *Three Part Breathing*

So often we find ourselves surprised, angry, or side-swiped when dealing with unexpected news. One of the healthiest ways to deal with change is to acknowledge that you feel unbalanced and see if you can reconnect with your internal GPS. Connecting with your breath will literally give you some breathing room before you open your mouth to say or do something you may regret. Give your body/mind a chance to go inside and recalibrate.

The following technique can be done in public or private. If you are standing or sitting in front of the bearer of the news, just soften your eyes and as quietly as possible say to yourself: *Inhale... Pause... Exhale... Pause.* If you are in private, in a bathroom, in the car by yourself, or taking a walk – it may be easier to say the words *inhale, pause,* and *exhale* out loud. It is often easier to do this exercise when you can really hear your breath. Always be respectful of your environment and the people who are nearby.

These techniques are meant to increase compassion and decrease any knee-jerk reaction that may cause more harm or add to the tension of the moment. If you are having trouble focusing, just name the situation or issue: Maybe the printer is jammed and you must get a document to someone as soon as possible: *Inhale printer, Pause, Exhale printer, Pause....* Maybe the car won't start: *Inhale car won't start, Pause, Exhale car won't start, Pause....* Maybe you are sitting in a doctor's office and have been waiting for over forty-five minutes: *Inhale waiting in the doctor's office, Pause, Exhale waiting in the doctor's office, Pause....* Maybe a loved one has just died. *Inhale person's name, Pause, Exhale person's name, Pause....* This deep breathing technique works for little, medium, and big issues. Think of something that is bugging you right now. Name it. Take a deep inhale as you name it, then pause, hold the situation in your mind's eye, and then on the next exhale let it go.

You may want to do several rounds of inhaling, pausing, exhaling and see if you can breathe some space into whatever you are dealing with in the moment. Breathing deeply and mindfully may not be an instant fix, but it will take the edge off the situation and give you some much needed time to recalibrate.

Inhale

Pause

Exhale

Pause

Inhale

Pause

Exhale

Pause

Inhale

Pause

Exhale

Pause

Inhale

Pause

Exhale

2. The Secret Power of the Pause

Many people think that the breath and breathing is simply an inhale and an exhale. Most of us miss the power of the *pause*. The *pause* offers us an opportunity to focus on linking our inhales and exhales. Think of it as the connector or a bridge between your inhale and your exhale. We usually get wrapped up in the inhale and the exhale; however the key here is taking time to really focus on the *pause*.

Most of us have experienced that feeling of having a "low battery," which often shows up as tiredness, fatigue, irritation, low energy, sleepiness, hunger, and even anger. If you want to recharge your batteries, you may want to experiment with paying attention to the *pause* between each inhale and exhale. Think of this as literally "pausing" your internal movie, DVD, or video. This is a wonderful technique to use to get your engine restarted and energize your body, mind, and spirit. It can also help you recalibrate as you move between tasks, emotions, situations, and transitions. It is also a great mini-meditation and mindfulness treat.

This technique may be challenging to incorporate into your everyday life; however, once you get it, it is like riding a bicycle – you will never lose it. You may even want to gradually work up to increasing the number of rounds. However, if you are forcing your body and/or your mind to do this, then you have missed the point of practicing true yoga.

On your next inhale, simply add a mindful *pause* before your exhale. And then *pause* before you take your next inhale. It really helps to literally say out loud: *inhale,* *pause, exhale,* *pause*.... I like to look for mini-opportunities throughout my day – like waiting for the kettle to boil in the kitchen, stuck at a stoplight, waiting for a ride, standing in line at the post office, being placed on hold on the phone, trying to go to sleep at night, waking up in the middle of the night – the list of opportunities is limitless.

*The Secret to Breathing Is Using the Pause Button**

Please

Pay

Attention

To

The

PAUSE

Between your

Inhale

and your

Exhale.

**The PAUSE is the secret for living
a juicier life regardless of how young you are.*

3. *Sealed with a Kiss*

Many of our ancestors believed that the spirit gods lived in the breath; hence, kisses were taken very seriously. Kisses were used to seal business deals, legal agreements, and marriage commitments; hence, the term "sealed with a kiss." In fact, the traditional words: "*You may now kiss the bride,*" are based on the ancient belief that we are offering our most precious gift to another person – our life force.

A wonderful way to use the power of your breath is to imagine that it is your spirit and that you can send it out into the universe to offer wellness and healing. Close your eyes and think of someone you know, someone who needs you, or it may even be someone you don't know. This image may be a family member or friend, or maybe a news photo of someone you may not know personally but for some reason that image resonates with you. It may also be a group of people or animals that are suffering. Picture this person or situation in your mind's eye for a few deep breaths.

On your next inhale, bring your hand to your lips, pause, and then as you exhale, kiss your fingertips. Then with your palm facing up toward the sky, gently blow that kiss from the tip of your fingertips out toward the person or situation in your mind's eye. See your breath flying through the universe and surrounding that person/situation with pure healing energy.

This is an incredibly healing mini-meditation and works on a family member, friend, or stranger who needs your help: "*I am sending you a blessing, wishing you a safe journey.*"

Choose words that resonate with you and not only will the receiver benefit, but so will you. You don't even have to do any hand motions or make any audible sounds. Simply visualize your breath and blessing moving outward toward your intention. I know this may sound a bit wacky – but it works. Try it!

4. *Heart Centered Breathing*

The yogis believe that the arms are an extension of the heart. So when you reach out to shake someone's hand or give him or her a hug – you are reaching out from your heart. Here are three variations of this heartfelt meditation:

a) **Hand to Heart Center**: Place your right or left hand on your chest between your breasts. Looking straight ahead, or down at your hand, eyes open or closed, begin to actively listen to your breathing. See if you can deepen and slow down your ***inhales*** and ***exhales***. Remember to ***pause*** between every inhale and exhale.

See if you can inhale the name of a person, place or thing that you're grateful for – it doesn't matter if this person is dead or alive. This practice may be done verbally or silently. I like to practice this exercise when I wake up in the morning, warm and snug in my bed. I usually start with inhaling/pausing/exhaling my gratitude for: *soft blankets, warm feet, chirping birds, a quiet house, coffee brewing...*

If I wake up in the middle of the night and can't go back to sleep, I usually start this practice with finding all the things to be grateful for, beginning with my *warm bed, clean sheets, stars outside the window...* and then I move on to *naming people who have helped me throughout my life – especially my family, friends, and relatives.* Again, it doesn't matter if they are dead or alive. Just place your hand between your breasts and *inhale, pause, exhale, pause...* as you name a specific gratitude or person.

This exercise also works if you are struggling with an issue, an uncomfortable emotion, or even a confrontation at home or in your workplace. See what happens when you name that situation on each *inhale, pause*, and *exhale*.

This breathing technique can often help you enter a challenging situation from the heart rather than from the mind. The mind sometimes gets in the way of our truthful heart.

b) **Hands to Heart Center**: This technique is similar to the above, except that both hands are pressed together as in a prayer position between your breasts. I sometimes like to place both hands flat on my chest, one over the other at my heart center. It usually takes me a few deep breaths before I can hear my heart beating. I can usually feel my blood pressure slowing down as my body totally relaxes.

I have noticed practicing this technique even for thirty seconds to a minute will make a difference before I go onto the next task. I like to close this mini-meditation by bringing my hands up to my lips and lightly kissing my fingertips. It's like blowing a kiss into your body.

Remember that you can do this anytime or anywhere – including lying down in bed, before you get out of your car, or anytime you need to recharge your batteries. It is also a good practice to do when you are thinking of someone who really could use your love and positive thoughts – including yourself!

c) **Licorice Ropes or How to Give Yourself a Hug**: Stretch both arms in front of you at shoulder level. Place your right wrist on top of your left wrist, roll your hands down toward each other and interlace your fingers. Keep your fingers interlaced as you drop your arms down and roll your hands towards your chest. Bring your licorice arms toward you until your hands are resting on your chest between your breasts. The arms, including your elbows, will naturally rest on your chest.

Please note that if you have arthritis, hand or shoulder issues, this movement may not be pleasurable and may not even be recommended. It is best to check with a health care practitioner. Always listen to your inner voice and never push through any pain. On the other hand, for many of us who are dealing with mild arthritis, this simple pretzel twist may increase our flexibility and elasticity. Whatever you do, be extremely gentle.

I like to spend at least thirty seconds to a few minutes on each side. This is an incredibly soothing and nurturing gesture. It can also be practiced when lying in bed. Be sure to do both sides – right wrist over left wrist and left wrist over right wrist!

d) How to Give Yourself a Hug: Place your right hand on your left shoulder and then your left hand on your right shoulder. Feel free to place your left hand on your right shoulder first and then the right hand on your left shoulder if that feels more comfortable and natural for you. Take a deep breath as you push the crown of the head up towards the sky. Feel your chest lift, let your breath pause and then exhale very slowly.

Give yourself a gentle shoulder squeeze with your hands and then release your hands to your sides.

It usually feels good to roll your shoulders back down and away from your ears; put some weight in the elbows and feel your chest broaden and your rib cage expand.

Remember to STOP if anything does NOT feel pleasurable and nurturing. And the icing on the cake is to find a person or animal, and give them a hug!

5. Breathing Meditation

There is a lot of talk in the news today about the benefits of meditation, including the evidence that it lowers blood pressure, relieves stress, slows down the aging process, benefits cardiovascular and immune health, and even improves concentration and brain function.

However, for some of us, meditation has just leaped onto our list of healthy habits we should be incorporating into our busy lives. Who has twenty minutes twice a day? Who has the discipline to do something regularly? I finally cracked the code on my reluctance to sit quietly twice a day by breaking the process down into bite-sized pieces. Here is how it works: I simply tell myself that I am going to take a few slow, deep breaths and if my mind wanders, I will simply go back to *inhale, pause, exhale, pause …*

Let's try it: Find a comfortable seat, you can even do this before you get out of bed in the morning! Take a deep long inhale, pause, and then take a long slow exhale. I like to say ONE before the first inhale and I use my fingers to keep count. You can also use a beaded bracelet, mala, or rosary. If you are sitting you can also use ten small rocks, coins, buttons, or paper clips. Get creative. Don't buy anything. You can move your meditation pieces onto a bowl or plate before or after every inhale or exhale. The key here is just focusing on the breath.

Here's the fun part: when you get to the tenth exhale YOU WILL WANT TO CONTINUE, because it feels so good. It's like coming into meditation/mindfulness through the back door. The body/mind/spirit loves this stuff, we did it naturally when we were infants. Think of it as home base. This is also a wonderful ritual to do between activities. And you don't need to use any props; simply look for opportunities to add a minute or two of meditation into your life. You can do this in your car, standing in line, waiting for class to start, sitting on the airplane during ascent or descent. Just do a few rounds of *inhale... pause... exhale... pause.* You will notice the more you add a few minutes of meditation throughout your day, the less stress will cling to you. Who knows, you may even get up to the recommended twenty minutes twice a day!

Food for Thought

The average person breathes in and out

up to 23,040 times a day.

However, most of us are not breathing very deeply

or mindfully.

ELEMENT TWO

Creating Internal Energy: Lifting the Spirit Within

Years ago, I read about an *aikido* master who could do amazing feats. He claimed that the secret was in his ability to use his breath to connect with his core. As a person who was raised on *"just try harder,"* this inner strength seemed very foreign to me until one day when I was hiking. The steep slope in front of me looked like it went straight up forever. I remembered one of the stories in that *aikido* book that described visualizing a rope attached to your belly just below your belly button, and if you looked ahead to where you wanted to go, you could just let the rope pull you towards your goal.

I relaxed and let the rope pull me up to the top of the hill. About five minutes later, my friends arrived, doubled over, panting, and asking how I *"sailed up the mountain."* To this day, if I am faced with a steep incline, I simply visualize that rope from the hike years ago pulling me up towards the top of the mountain.

The take-home here is that when we stop, relax, breathe, and have a clear goal, we will get there much faster.

Isometric lifts are a fantastic way to strengthen your core muscles, lift your diaphragm, and improve your posture. These movements are also known as static strength training because there is no visible movement in the joints.

The best way to describe an internal lift is to try the following: *Rest your hand gently on your belly button; now without moving your hand, see if you can pull your belly button towards your spine.* The following movements are often subtle, however you will find over time that they will give you amazing internal core strength. If you have any physical issues, including recent abdominal surgery, or experience any pain with any of these postures, please review them with your health care practitioner.

Yoga Rx:
Creating Internal Energy

1. **Lifting the Sky**

2. **Strengthening the Pelvic Floor**

3. **Hand Springs**

4. **Chin to Chest**

5. **Internal Visualizations**

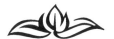

1. *Lifting the Sky*

Lifting the Sky is a simple movement that not only expands your chest and helps you to breathe deeper, it elongates the body and feels absolutely empowering.

You can do this movement sitting down or standing up; however, the best way to get a sense of this is to stand up, and then without moving your feet, see if you can gently push the crown of your head up towards the sky.

At the same time, feel your chest lifting, your rib cage and lungs expanding, your shoulders dropping away from your ears. This always gives me a sense of elongation – as if I just grew two inches. I like to practice this whenever I am walking or standing in line or just find myself collapsing with the weight of the world on my shoulders.

Once you get the hang of this, you can do it while sitting down in a chair. It will also assist in relieving fatigue by giving your lungs a chance to expand and get a boost of oxygen. I always feel more open, loving, and happy whenever I remember to "lift the sky!"

2. Strengthening the Pelvic Floor

What if you had to urinate and I told you that the next bathroom stop was three hours away? You may want to practice this ancient yoga technique, called *mulabundha*. It may be practiced standing, sitting, or even lying down in bed. It is basically isolating the perineal muscle, the area between the genitals and the anus. In females, it is the perineum muscle at the top of the cervix. It is often comparable to doing pelvic floor exercises or *Kegels.* Men can also use this technique to strengthen the urinary sphincter.

A convenient place to practice this is when you are going to the bathroom; just hold your urine mid-stream for a second, then release. Be sure NOT to tense the muscles in your buttocks, legs or abdomen, or hold your breath. When you slow or stop the flow of urine, you've successfully engaged these muscles. Be sure to start slowly and never push yourself. You may feel awkward at first, but after a while you will notice that your pelvic floor muscles are stronger and you may even find yourself feeling more centered and standing up taller.

The good news is that you can do this contraction anytime and anywhere, no one will see you. As you inhale, pause, and gently contract the urinary muscles, pause, and then as you exhale, slowly release and relax those muscles. If you forget to do it at random times during the day, just do it every time you urinate. This internal lift will not only strengthen your pelvic floor, it will tone your inner core and elongate your torso, and it does wonders for your posture.

3. Hand Springs

Before you run out and buy a set of hand grippers or exercise squeeze balls, I suggest you to try this exercise. On your next inhale, make two fists with your hands and squeeze your fists as tightly as you can. Then as you exhale, slowly unclench your fists, and stretch your fingers open as widely as they will go today. *Did you feel a bit of a tingle? A bit of pressure released?*

The next time you are feeling stressed about something, simply inhale and squeeze your fingers into the palms of your hands. Make two fists, hold as tightly as you can for a second or two, and then release your fists on an exhale. Sometimes it helps to name the issue or person as you inhale on a squeeze. You may want to do this several times, depending on the severity of whatever is causing your body to tense or your blood pressure to rise.

Sometimes just taking a minute to squeeze and release any tension will give you a mini *timeout,* and an opportunity to pause and take a deep breath. You may even come up with a solution to your situation.

When I started researching hand grippers for building hand strength, I was amazed at the options of grippers, squeeze balls, digit-flex hand/finger exercises, gel handballs, and foam hand exercisers (that can be used in warm, hot, or cold water). They come in various sizes, weights, and tensions. Before you go out and purchase a hand gripper, you may want to do some research, including consulting a physical/occupational therapist, body trainer, or health care practitioner.

Remember you do not need to be a rock climber, athlete, or body builder to benefit from increasing hand and arm strength. These exercises will give you more hand and finger flexibility, coordination, dexterity, mobility, and forearm strength. Who knows, they may even help you open those pickle jars!

4. Chin to Chest

This simple posture always reminds me that even small movements done throughout the day can help release tension and stress before it develops into a more intense issue.

On your next inhale, pause, and then as you exhale, drop your chin towards your chest. Continue breathing gently and remember that this is not about squeezing your chin to your chest and creating more stress; it's all about using your heavy head to release any tension in the back of the neck and the shoulder area.

For an additional stretch, you may want to pull your shoulders down, away from your ears. This helps release neck and shoulder tension. Be sure to proceed slowly and gently, especially if you have had any neck or shoulder injuries or surgeries. Practicing these movements will also help you to stand or sit up straighter. The most important thing is to keep breathing and relax into the posture for as long as it feels good.

Sometimes I like to place my hands in a prayer position, palms pressed together with my thumbs resting on my chest between my breasts. This is an excellent time to say a prayer, do a mini-meditation, or simply look down at your fingertips and thank your beautiful hands for all the work they do. Remember to back off if there is any discomfort or pain in your neck and shoulders.

5. *Internal Visualizations*

Did you know that when we are in pain we tend to hold our breath? The next time you are dealing with an injury – whether it is physical or emotional – you may like to try this internal visualization. Close your eyes or leave them slightly open. Take a few slow deep breaths, being mindful to pause between your inhales and your exhales. Then move your breath to the part of your body that hurts; it may be your big toe, a knee joint, or a broken heart. The key here is to FOCUS on your injury. See if you can inhale your pain, pause, and then as you exhale – release your pain. I find this exercise easier to do when I actually name the body part or the person that is bothering me out loud. This is not an instant fix; however, it can be incredibly soothing and comforting.

The other side of the coin is to NOT focus on your pain. If you are in an uncomfortable place, like squished into an airline seat, waiting in a physician's office, or about to walk into a potentially volatile meeting, see if you can take your mind to a beautiful setting. Sometimes just visualizing your favorite place in nature will give you a stress-free mini-vacation and an opportunity to totally relax! In other words, daydream! Make up a great story and go there. Either way the discomfort or pain may still exist, but you will notice that either method will often relax the body, take the edge off the situation, and lift your spirits.

Food for Thought

There is a voice that doesn't use words. Listen.

— Rumi

ELEMENT THREE

Gazing In & Out: Connecting the Inside with the Outside

Years ago one of my yoga teachers told me this story. He was in a car crash, hospitalized and put into traction, unable to move his arms and legs. Yet he continued to practice his yoga. He simply visualized his favorite yoga postures whenever he was awake. Six weeks later, his physicians and therapists took all the casts off and watched in amazement as he returned very closely to his pre-accident range of motion and flexibility.

Olympic athletes – in football, tennis, basketball, hockey, volleyball, golf, skiing – pre-visualize the event that they are approaching, including possible obstacles. So when they hit a bump in the road their body/mind has already anticipated it and they can respond quickly. The good news is that you don't have to be a professional athlete to use this powerful tool.

Visualizations can strengthen the mind and also can be practiced as a form of meditation. Some people would label my flights of fancy as daydreaming. All I know is that I find it absolutely relaxing and fun to do athletic feats I would never do in my everyday life. I am not a skier, but in my mind I can visualize a helicopter dropping me off at the top of a mountain, before I ski down steep slopes. I am not a skater, but I can do a triple Lutz in my mind. This internal practice is really relaxing and you may even discover something interesting about yourself.

There is a beautiful Sanskrit word, *drishti,* which is often translated as *focus or gazing points.* It usually refers to where our eyes are looking or what we are focusing on. Gazing points are often used in yoga postures to help you balance and move between poses. These focus points also may be used as a meditation technique such as *gazing at the tip of your nose, a sacred object, your hands in prayer position, or focusing internally at a point between your eyebrows.* Most of us have had the experience of gazing deeply into the eyes of someone we love – a spouse, parent, friend, child – even a dog or cat. It is the feeling that Martin Buber stated so beautifully in the experience of a loving *I–Thou* relationship: "*I see you and you see me. We are one.*"

I am not recommending that you gaze deeply into everyone's eyes, however it is helpful to notice what catches your gaze and how you use your eyes throughout the day. You may also practice looking deep into your own eyes in the bathroom mirror. What comes up for you? Is it awkward? Are you gazing with love into your reflection or are you criticizing the reflection? It is also a healthy practice to notice your surroundings: take a moment right now and look up from this page. What is the first thing that catches your eye?

Yoga Rx:
Gazing In & Out

1. **Director: Starring in Your Own Movie**

2. **Hands on the Wheel**

3. **Eye Care**

4. **Seeing TRUTH**

5. **Climbing Your Own Mt. Everest**

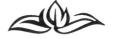

1. Director:
Starring in Your Own Movie

Pretend that you are a movie director filming yourself. This may feel awkward at first, however it can be fun, interesting, and very revealing. Start with brushing your teeth. Just pretend that you are being filmed while brushing your teeth. You may find yourself standing up a bit straighter and smiling into the mirror.

Or you may want to pretend that you are demonstrating how to make a bed, do laundry, or make a salad. This is simply a technique to make you more mindful as you go about your daily tasks. In fact, it usually cheers me up because I become more aware of how important it is to stand up straight and smile as I go about my day.

If no one is around, I sometimes talk to myself or pretend that I am doing a voiceover describing what I am doing. Practicing this technique has given me a chance to slow down and experience gratitude for so many things that I take for granted. When was the last time you thanked the hot water coming out of the bathroom faucet?

2. Hands on the Wheel

Most of us are usually so busy multitasking that we often miss opportunities to create little meditations. In fact, most of us have had the experience of driving to work, an appointment, or a restaurant, so wrapped up in some drama in our head that when we get out of the car, we can't even remember how we got to the parking lot!

The next time you find your mind wandering – whether you are traveling by bicycle, car, bus, subway, or train – you may want to try the following. As the driver, your internal dialog may go something like this: *Hands on the wheel at ten and two o'clock, picking up the car key, inserting it in the key slot and turning the key, engine engaging, check mirror, putting car in reverse, backing up slowly…*

If you are the passenger, your internal dialog may go something like this: *Putting on the seatbelt, checking to make sure my water bottle is secure, kicking my shoes off, adjusting seat position, great view out window, love the light on that tree…*

You can create mini-meditations throughout your busy day by focusing on the actual moment and NOT thinking about WHERE you are going or WHAT you are going to do when you get to your destination. The next time you are traveling in a vehicle or even walking, see if you can describe exactly what you are seeing. If this is difficult, pretend that you are telling a blind person what you are seeing. Notice what happens to your body, mind, and mood.

3. Eye Care

Have you ever stopped to record how much time you spend staring at a digital screen? Many of us today are frequent users of computers, cell phones, tablets, televisions, e-readers, and some of us are literally plugged in all day. Most of us are unaware of how much time we spend on our electronic devices until the electricity goes off, the internet is down, we are out of cell range, or we have had eye surgery. How often do we gaze out the window and really look at a tree, a bird in flight, or a dog running around? Here are a few suggestions on how to rest your eyes during the day:

a) **Take frequent breaks away from your electronic devices:** Get up and go get a glass of water or do a few stretches. Take a deep breath, shrug your shoulders up to your ears, do neck rolls and stretch your arms overhead. Even just standing up on your tippy toes and doing some calf stretches will help to release tension in your body. Be sure to blink your eyes and let them rest on something that is not electronic or digital. You may even want to create an electronic reminder to rest your eyes throughout the day!

b) **Close Your Eyes:** If you are wearing glasses, set them down in a safe place before closing your eyes. If you are wearing contacts be very mindful not to squeeze your eyelids too tightly. Just keep your eyes gently closed for a few breaths. Continue to take a few deep breaths and see if you can soften and relax the forty-three-plus muscles in your face. I like to close my eyes and just listen. How many sounds can I identify? When you open your eyes you may find your vision has improved. And who knows, you may even be smiling!

c) **Clock Face:** If you are wearing glasses, set them down in a safe place. If you are wearing contacts, be very mindful of any discomfort. Soften your eyes and pretend that you are facing a giant clock face. Roll your eyes straight up to twelve o'clock and then continue to take your eyes to the right going clockwise counting very slowly through each hour and winding back at twelve o'clock. I find it easier to focus when I count out loud. Then reverse your eye rolls, going counter-clockwise from twelve o'clock through each hour until you are back to twelve o'clock. I find that when I go as slowly as I can, taking deep inhales and exhales, my entire body feels much more relaxed. Sometimes I do several rotations as a mini-meditation session. It also feels good to close your eyes for a few deep breaths before going back to your busy day.

d) **Sunglasses:** When outside on a sunny day, even in the winter, be sure to protect your eyes with sunglasses. It's not just the UV rays shining directly or indirectly into our eyes, but we need to protect the delicate area around the eyes and eyelids. According to eye doctors, seven to ten percent of all skin cancers are found on the eyelid. Even our eyes can get sunburnt, leading to increased eye pain, blurry vision, and the sensation of having sand in your eye. The shorter the wavelength, the more harmful the UV radiation. Be sure to pick up a pair of sunglasses that block UVA and UVB light. If you have any questions, please discuss this with your eye doctor or physician at your next checkup.

e) **Safety Glasses:** The best way to avoid an accident is to take safety precautions. Not only do ice hockey players, welders, and tree trimmers need to protect their eyes – we all do. It's a good idea to be pro-active and wear your regular glasses or clear safety glasses with side shields when doing yard work and doing heavy cleaning with lots of dust or chemicals. Taking care of yourself includes working with a buddy and having your cell phone nearby.

Rx for Ladder Safety

ALWAYS have someone with you, or better yet, get someone much younger and more agile than you to do anything that involves climbing and/or a ladder; it is not worth falling. And if you don't believe me ask anyone over sixty years young if they know anyone who has fallen off a ladder, suffered physically, and/or died due to complications and injuries from a fall. It is simply not worth the risk.

4. *Seeing TRUTH*

Stop lying. We all lie. Even a white lie is still a lie. Can you experiment and see if you can go all day without telling any lies? How about we just start with the next hour? What happens when you hold yourself to speaking only the truth? I am not advocating that you be rude about telling someone they are annoying, sloppy, or mean. I am simply asking us to start looking within and see if we can start by telling the truth to ourselves. Can we practice the art of pausing before we lie to ourselves and others? Isn't it just better to say: *I am not hungry, I am upset. I can't stay up late, it just doesn't work for me. Is there a matinee? I'd love to do dinner, but your spouse's politics upset me; can you and I just take a walk or visit over a cup of tea?*

What is truth? It is the actual state of a matter, a fact that can be verified and involves honesty and integrity. Can we just state the facts? *My hair flips up on one side and down on the other... I always have more than one cookie... I don't like people who disagree with me.* When I state the truth, it doesn't hurt as much. It takes all the spin and song and dance out of my issues. My hair never looks like the magazine photos. I love cookies and rarely eat just one. I have to take a really deep breath when I run into people I disagree with. I need to separate the person from the issue and find some common ground.

The above issues may be petty on the scale of worldwide angst, but I have found that the more I deal with my truths in my daily interactions, the more aware I am of when I am not living my truths. We get into trouble if we do not stay open to the truth. It can reside deep inside of us and can keep us away from living a more joyful life. It can be stressful to be open to hearing the truth, changing our point of view, or realizing that we may not have the whole story. However, like any other good habit, it is worth it!

One way to get in touch with your truth is to name your core values and use them to actively evaluate your interactions with the world. The key is pausing before you pass judgement on something you have heard or read. Before you totally believe a news release, you may want to consider the source and do some research. The same goes for receiving a tasty tidbit of gossip: is it vital to pass along? And instead of complaining about your daughter-in-law to everyone, why not figure out how to communicate with her, let it go, or get creative about taking care of yourself without contributing to more family strife?

We have a policy where I work called the *24-Hour Rule.* You have 24 hours to get back to the person who ruffled your feathers and deal with it. Your complaints expire in 24 hours. We also discourage triangulation. When a co-worker complains about another co-worker to me, I immediately suggest they talk to that person directly. My co-workers do the same for me when I am complaining or upset about someone's actions or non-actions. I have also learned to use this technique in communicating with my family and friends. If I have an issue with my spouse, I do not complain to my sister about him, I go directly to my spouse to discuss the issue or I drop it.

The more you practice telling the truth to yourself, the more sensitive you will become to perceiving lies, fabricated stories, and misleading sound bites. You will find your-self feeling lighter for being more candid, transparent, and honest with yourself. This includes NOT sharing everything. Sometimes silence and letting things go is the high road. You will find that by keeping your own personal slate as clean as possible, you will have more time and energy for the people you love and hopefully leave the world a better place.

5. *Climbing Your Own Mt. Everest*

If you are over fifty years old, you most likely have a list of *should have, could have, would have* regrets from your past. This is also known as *shoulda, coulda, woulda*. The good news is that we have an opportunity to honestly examine our past and move on. This is not about wishing something were different; this is all about seeing if you have any pebbles of regret in your shoes that need to be dealt with. We all have regrets, this is just a wake-up call to be honest and see if there is something in your past that would feel good to get out in the open and resolve.

This may involve asking for forgiveness from someone who is still alive or even someone who has died. It may involve writing a letter, mailing it or shredding it, or simply telling yourself you did the best you could under the circumstances. Take a few minutes to honestly look at yourself and see if there is still something that needs to be done or accomplished before your die. I call this: *Climbing Your Own Mt. Everest*. Will you regret not accomplishing this task, item and/or conversation on your deathbed? Take the next few days to really think, write, draw, walk, talk, and see what comes up for you. Ask yourself the following questions:

a) **Do I need to do anything before dying** concerning my friends, family, education, career, parenting, marriage, relationships, finances, home/house, projects, travels, creativity, advanced directives, estate or will? Do not stop and judge how small, petty, or big some of these mountains are. Simply take note and don't panic if the task seems daunting. The answers on how to resolve the situation will come to you.

b) **Is there an issue that I need to complete in order to die in peace?** Imagine you just found out that you are going to die tomorrow morning. *What angst is left on your plate?* Is there any issue, person, or incident that is still bothering you right now? How important is it that you resolve it? What can you let go of, and what can you change? Are you holding on to any lies of omission? Are you NOT telling the truth, when it would make a positive change for the better? This is often an uncomfortable place, however the truth will set you free.

c) **What can I do right now to start Climbing My Own Mt. Everest?** I have met many people in the hospice program who were in pain over unsaid things, especially to loved ones. Or they were carrying around a major regret over something they really wanted to do but for whatever reason, never completed. Maybe you literally wanted to climb Mt. Everest, sky dive in Mexico, or go to Bali, but now your health issues have prevented it. Get creative. There is always a solution, including funding someone else's dream to climb a mountain, jump out of an airplane, or go to Indonesia. We may continue to live our dreams through our gifts and legacy to others. Yes, it may be extra work, time and money, however I can tell you from my personal experience, it is worth the peace and equanimity you will receive in return.

Food for Thought

Your vision will become clear only

when you look into your own heart.

Who looks outside – dreams.

Who looks inside – awakens.

— C.G. Jung

ELEMENT FOUR

Movement 24/7: Anytime & Anywhere

One day I woke up late and realized that I had no time to do my usual yoga routine if I was going to get to work on time. So I decided to see if I could work some yoga postures into my day using whatever was right in front of me as a prop. My first posture I called *Microwave Yoga*. Instead of just standing motionless waiting for my coffee to reheat, I took a deep breath and pretended I was standing on my yoga mat. I stretched my arms overhead and did two delicious stretches – thirty seconds on each side. I was thrilled! I felt great. I couldn't believe how simply and easily two stretches could be incorporated into my everyday routine. Instead of being pissed off all day because I missed my morning stretch routine, I spent the rest of the day looking for opportunities to *do some yoga postures* without being on my yoga mat!

Definition of a Yoga Posture

The word *asana* usually brings up images of perfect yoga postures performed by the buff models on the cover of a yoga magazine. I prefer to use the ancient definition of a yoga posture (*Asana*) as in a "comfortable seat" (*Patanjali*). So if I am sitting straight up at my desk, totally centered, breathing and pain free – I am in a yoga posture.

Definition of Movement

The dictionary definition of *movement* is very broad. It can mean anything from an activity to the appearance of motion as in a painting or sculpture; a political action group; a change in the market price of a security or a commodity; or simply the evacuation of the bowels! *Yoga* is all about focusing on *movement* as in physically moving our bodies, including our bowels. I like to avoid the word *exercise,* simply because for me, it usually conjures up a sense of dread, heaviness or guilt, as in: *I know I really should exercise more often... My doctor told me to take this exercise class... I'm too tired to go for a walk today... I am too stuffed from last night's dinner to exercise this morning... I'm too fat... Why bother, I am going to die anyway...*

Your homework today is to replace the word *exercise* with the word *movement* and look for opportunities throughout your day to add a stretch. If you need inspiration, just watch a cat, dog or child move, and imitate them. I guarantee you will feel instantly lighter, happier, and more optimistic.

The best way to look at movement is that you are investing in your personal healthy body savings account. Every action, including sitting still in meditation or prayer, is a positive step towards living a fuller and juicier life. Begin right now in the very next breath to give your body the love, care, and support it deserves.

I hope the following ideas will inspire you to look around your environment for more opportunities to consciously add more movement to your day.

NOTE: *If you haven't been physically moving for a while and/or are recovering from a surgery, illness, or injury – please start ANY new movement slowly. There is no reason to put further stress on your body. Start by taking baby steps while always treating yourself with loving kindness. Listening to your body will help you avoid injuries, and help you build and maintain strength. Please remember that even if you have a chronic condition, are in a convalescent home, or are recovering from surgery – you can still practice yoga breathing!*

Yoga Rx: Moving 24/7

1. **Getting Clear on Why You Want to Be Healthy**

2. **Microwave Yoga: Creating a Home Studio/Gym/Workout Space**

3. **Riding the Tube: Mouth to Bowels**

4. **Moving Assets: Spring Cleaning Year Around**

5. **Practicing Stillness: Doing Nothing**

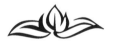

1. Why Bother? Getting Clear on Why You Want to Be Healthy

The challenge that we all face in creating a healthy life-style is the realization that we will eventually die. If you do not understand **why** you are choosing healthy movement versus: "*Why bother, I am going to die anyway,*" then you will be like the dieters who lose a bunch of weight and then gain it back. Many dieters do not address the core reason **why** they were overweight in the first place. What are we looking for in that bag of cookies, chips, or bagels? Love? Security? Acknowledgment? Peace? Touch? Sex? Our body/weight issues are as multifaceted as our reasons for not creating opportunities to move our bodies.

Animals and children do this well, they move their bodies for sheer pleasure. They are constantly releasing tension and stress by letting it out through their bodies, and sometimes their lungs! Why are we avoiding our bodies?

Take a good honest look at why you want to stay healthy. There is no *right* answer here, only *your* answer. Your answer does not have to be set in stone. Our life changes; we need to be able to readjust as our circumstances change. The only advice I can offer here is to start moving right now. Put down this book and move. Do some neck rolls, scrunch your face into a prune or a raisin face, wiggle your toes, squeeze your hands into fists on an inhale, and open them wide on an exhale, or get down on the floor and stretch like a cat. Now how do you feel?

If you are not sure why you are still living, or what the purpose of the remainder of your life is, it's time to take an honest look. A good place to start is to ask yourself: *What gives me pleasure?*

Another way to look at this is to notice what you will miss when you are dead. This may include friends, family, grandchildren, animals, chocolate croissants, Earl Grey tea, sunrise, sunset, music, reading, sewing, baking, entertaining, playing Scrabble, traveling – *your list will be different from my list*. There may even be a surprise or two. The whole idea is to focus your time and attention on what really matters to you and let go of the people, activities, and issues that drain your energy and/or no longer give you pleasure. The bottom line is that this is your life and you are responsible for honoring your body, mind, and spirit from this day forward.

The Joy and Pleasure List

There will always be chores in our life, even getting out of bed in the morning when we've had a rough night can be difficult. And then there is the image of our youth: all the activities and things that we could do in one day are no longer realistic. Instead of being depressed and upset: why not shift your energy? Before we go any further, write down ten activities that you love to do. No one pays you to do these things, you do them simply because they give you pleasure and joy.

Here's a sample of my list today (it changes with the seasons):

1. Reading books and magazines.
2. Walking by myself or with a friend.
3. Calling a good friend or family member just because I am thinking about them.

4. Writing or drawing in my journal or sketchbook.

5. Napping (with a book or a cup of tea).

6. Sending notes to friends and family via email or snail mail.

7. Giving something away. I always keep a donation box in the garage.

8. Making a cup of tea or coffee.

9. Rearranging a drawer or closet space.

10. Sitting and staring out the window. Watching birds, squirrels, or even just staring at the clouds in the sky is especially relaxing.

NOTE: *When you finish writing your list, choose one activity and do it right now. Be sure to do at least one thing on your joy and pleasure list every day.*

Food for Thought

What is on your pleasure list? Can you stop reading and write down ten activities that give you joy and pleasure? Is there something on that list that you can stop and do right now? Remember that this is NOT a bucket list of things you would like to do. You can still write down travel, which may include a travel video, hearing about a friend's cruise or kayak trip, reading a travel book or combining your love of food into a culinary tour of a country you are interested in. Travel may even include taking a bus ride to the next town and going to a new restaurant or museum. And if making the bed, washing clothes, or cleaning the sink gives you pleasure – put it on your list. Remember everyone will have a different list. You may even notice that on your "good days" you will have done several activities on your list. That's why it's important to incorporate your joy and pleasure list into your daily life.

2. *Microwave Yoga*

The idea behind *Microwave Yoga* is to find time to add movement into your everyday life. I am not suggesting that this would replace your regular exercise classes. I am simply encouraging you to look for hidden opportunities to use your home or workplace as a studio or gym. One of my friends calls this *furniture yoga* because beds, chairs, and tables make great yoga props! For the next few weeks as you move through your daily activities, slow down and pretend that you are a physical therapist or exercise physiologist looking for opportunities to turn your home/workplace into a mini-studio/gym.

If you need some ideas, here is a list of possibilities that I use at home, in the office, and when traveling. Feel free to borrow, modify, or expand on any of the following ideas. I have not put repetitions on each movement because I want to make sure that you customize them to fit your needs. Remember to always be aware of creating a safe space around you so that you do not injure yourself. If something does not feel right, or you experience any sharp pain, ***please back off immediately***. These movements are supposed to give you pleasure, not cause further pain or harm.

WARNING:

Beware of Wearing Socks Without Shoes.

Whenever You Do Any Movement,

Please Wear Firm Shoes or Go Barefoot!

a) **The Kitchen** offers a great workout option! It's easy to do a few stretches while you are waiting for the kettle to boil, the coffeemaker to brew, or the microwave to ping. (Please note: If you have any cardiovascular issues, please check with your health practitioner to make any necessary modifications to the following stretches.)

- My all-time favorite stretch is *picking apples.* Simply stretch your arms overhead, reach up and start "picking apples." Your hands will get an extra squeeze as you wrap your hand around the "apple" and then reach up with the other hand and pick another "apple." Be careful not to reach up too high; you want to feel a slight stretch on each side of your rib cage, not a rip and a tear. Just reach up as high as feels comfortable today.

- Another variation of the above stretch is *swaying palm trees* or *bamboo in the wind.* Begin by stretching your arms up over your head with your palms facing each other. It's OK if you don't get your arms up all the way – shoulder level works too. Just think Saguaro cactus with arms out at right angles.

- Again, if you experience any joint/shoulder pain, do not do this stretch. I like to use my breath as I inhale my arms up, pause, exhale as I bend to the right and pause, inhale up to center, pause, and exhale as I bend gently to the left, pause, and then inhale back to center. You want to go just far enough to feel a pleasurable stretch. Anything deeper that will cause pain defeats the whole purpose of moving gently.

- Kitchen counters are great for extra support as you stand on one leg and then the other. Think *flamingo standing on one leg* as you hold on to the edge of the counter. You can also lean up against the kitchen sink and lift one foot at a time off the floor one or two inches. And then remember to do the other side. You can also use a kitchen or dining room chair for support.

b) **Chair Squats**: This is sometimes used as an assessment tool for assisted living facilities to analyze a person's risk for falling. The good news is that you can start today to strengthen your thigh muscles at home. Begin by simply finding a firm chair that has a straight back and no wheels. Place the chair against the wall or the edge of the kitchen/dining room table with the seat facing out. Adjust your feet away from the edge of the chair so that when you sit down your buttocks land on the front edge of the chair. I like to have my feet hip-width apart for stability.

- Take a few deep breaths and on the next exhale, slowly lower your buttocks down to the edge of the chair, pause, and on an inhale, press your feet into the floor, and lift back up to a standing position. Be sure to keep your knees over your ankles, and let your weight settle into your heels. Sometimes it helps to have your arms out in front of you for balance, or you can place another chair in front of you with the back of the chair facing you so that you have something to hold onto.

- Remember to start slowly. You might only do one chair squat today, but look around your home. I am guessing that if you do one squat each time you walked by a firm chair you would have strengthened your thighs without additional hours in the gym.

c) **Stretching in Bed:** The following movements are easier to do lying on your back on a firm mattress or on a well-carpeted floor.

- Starting with your feet, point your feet away from your face, and then flex your toes towards your face. You can also slide your heels away from you towards the foot of the bed to get an even deeper stretch. Experiment by stretching one leg at a time, and then both legs simultaneously.

- Rest your heels on the mattress or the floor with your toes pointing straight up in the air, and then move your feet like windshield wipers from side to side. You can even get creative and move your right and left foot in different directions. Your brain will thank you for the workout!

- As you move your awareness up your legs, see if you can squeeze your thighs as you inhale, pause, and then on an exhale release them. Do this several times and your standing squats will become easier.

- Place your hands on your belly button, inhale, pause, and then on your next exhale pull your belly button towards your spine, pause, and inhale as the belly rises and softens. This meditative sequence is excellent for calming your emotions and relaxing the entire body. It is also a good practice if you are really upset about something or have insomnia.

- Place one or both hands between your breasts at your heart center, and take several deep slow breaths, remembering to *pause* between each inhale and each exhale. You will feel your entire body slowly start to relax.

- If you have a sore throat pending, or have emotional issues brewing, you may want to experiment with placing one hand gently on your throat, and repeat the breathing sequence above. There is something incredibly healing about combining your breath with your touch.

- At any time during the day, if your hands are clean, rub them together briskly until they are really warm, and then release your hands, and place them gently over your eyes. (Be sure to take your eyeglasses off; and if you are wearing contacts, be careful.) Rest your fingertips lightly on your forehead and the palms of your hands on your cheeks. Make sure that there is absolutely no pressure on the eyes. As your hands cool, simply release your arms to your side and enjoy that feeling of your face softening. Extra credit for smiling!

- You can even dance in bed! See if you can wiggle your arms and legs, and do all sorts of crazy poses. Dancing is great for stimulating blood flow (and since you are totally supported by the mattress, you don't have to worry about falling). This is a wonderful way to start or end your day.

d) **Brushing Your Teeth:** Place your weight on one leg as you lift the other leg up an inch off the floor. You may also lean on the sink for additional support. If you have an electric toothbrush, you can use the timer for giving each side equal opportunity. Don't forget to look in the mirror and notice your shoulders. Are you scrunching your shoulders up by your ears to compensate for your one-legged stance? Gently pull those shoulders down and away from your ears. You will find that by expanding your chest you will be able to breathe better. I don't recommend standing on one leg when flossing, I've tried it. I need both feet on the floor when I floss.

e) **Toilet Quads:** Getting up and down from the toilet offers a wonderful opportunity to work on your thigh muscles. See if you can engage the quads by squeezing your thighs as you slowly lower your buttocks down to rest on the toilet seat. When you are ready to stand back up, place both feet firmly on the floor, and press back up into a standing position. If you have a grab bar, you can incorporate it by slowly loosening your grip as you get stronger. Be sure to focus on what you are doing in the moment by moving slowly and mindfully. And always choose safety over pushing your limits. Falling, especially in the bathroom, may lead to more serious issues.

f) **Washing Hands:** Washing your hands is a healthy habit; however, most of us do not do a very thorough job. Washing your hands can offer you a gratitude, mindfulness, or mini-meditation opportunity. I have found that singing or humming the *Happy Birthday* song, not only gives me time to apply soap and lather the backs of my hands, between my fingers, and under my fingernails but it also makes me smile! You can sing any song, say a prayer, chant a mantra – anything that works for you. This is also a wonderful opportunity to add a little hand cream as you dry your hands. You can give yourself a hand massage and take a moment to sincerely thank your hands for taking care of yourself and your loved ones all these years.

g) **Socks:** Putting on your socks offers a perfect opportunity to work on your balance. The goal here is to stand on one foot as you lift the other foot up and put your sock on. For most of us this can be extremely challenging, especially if we are thinking about something else, have trouble with balancing, or have any knee or hip joint issues.

- Start by sitting on the edge of a chair or on the side of the bed. This is a good time to point and flex your toes. If your ankles are stable, you may want to add some ankle rolls. You may even want to take a minute to massage your feet with a light cream or lotion. When you are ready to put your socks on, see if you can add some leg lifts or stretches. You may want to experiment with stretching your leg out in front of you as you point and flex your feet. I like to put my hands under my thighs for extra support.

- Whatever you do, always move slowly, gently, and let your breath be your guide. If you are feeling stable, then move to a standing position. Start with leaning on your dresser as you put your socks on one at a time. If you are feeling stronger, then move away from any support.

SAFETY TIP: *When I am putting my socks on, I always have my back to the bed just in case I fall. Then I have a great cushion if I do fall! Always be careful. Socks have a nasty way of causing us to slip and fall, so please remember that safety is always the first defense in avoiding injuries.*

h) **Talking on the Phone**: I usually do not recommend multi-tasking, but this seems to be a good time to use your phone conversations to work out some physical kinks and keep your body juicy. Adding movement is useful if you are put on hold. I highly recommend wearing a headset or putting your phone on speaker mode. Be sure to tell the other person that they are on speaker-phone. This makes it easier to take notes, draw, or walk around.

- If you have complete privacy, simply sit on the floor with your back against the wall or door. Legs can be crossed or straight out in front of you. Be sure to have a chair nearby if getting up and down from the floor is challenging for you.

- You may also choose to sit on a firm chair to practice some chair yoga, chair squats, or leg lifts while talking on the phone.

The ideas above are only the tip of the iceberg. There are endless variations and opportunities for you to keep your body, mind, and spirit flexible. Simply taking a deep breath in, pausing, and then exhaling slowly as you roll your shoulders down and away from your ears is a yoga movement! If you continue to incorporate movement throughout your day, I guarantee you will feel better, lighter, and happier. Remember to have fun, get creative, and see how you can use objects in your home and your office to add some movement to your life.

3. Riding the Tube: Mouth to Bowels

We seniors may joke about our bowel movements, but it is comforting to know that the ancient yogis were very aware of the importance of cleaning all their bodily holes, from *neti* pots for their noses, homemade toothbrushes for their teeth, tongue scrapers for minimizing oral bacteria, drinking lots of water to clear their intestines, and even using moving water to cleanse their bowels in streams and rivers. I am not going to go into enemas, the color of your stools, or how much your poop should float. However, as the spouse of a dentist, I also have been a longtime advocate of finding the magic foods that will give me gorgeous white teeth, great digestion, and a constipation/diarrhea/burp/fart-free lifestyle. This is what I have learned: *It all starts in the mouth!*

NOTE: *If you have any gastrointestinal issues, please consult your health care practitioner.*

Fiberlicous!

Want to live healthier and lighter? Then slowly increase your fiber intake. Take a close look at what you are eating. If you really want to get serious, keep a food diary or a log. There is a significant fiber difference between drinking a glass of apple juice and eating an apple, munching processed vegetable chips and eating a bowl of chopped vegetables, or eating a small piece of chicken or a big bowl of chicken soup.

Which food will fill you up more and last longer: a handful of potato chips or a plain baked potato? I am NOT saying never eat processed food. I am saying give your body an internal cleanse by eating real food with real fiber. Your gut will thank you in the long run!

NOTE: *Fiber comes in two forms – soluble and insoluble. Some foods have both forms. Think of fiber as little brushes whisking the walls of your intestinal tract and keeping everything moving briskly down the tube. The good news is that if you are eating at least five servings of fresh fruits, vegetables, and some grain products every day, you are probably meeting your daily fiber requirement.*

If you have any questions about the amount of fiber you need, please consult your health care practitioner. The internet offers some excellent lists of fiber content of different foods. Please be cautious of any company trying to sell you magic pills, elixirs, or stool cleanses in exchange for your credit card number. Many over-the-counter products are just bulk psyllium seed husks wrapped in shiny paper.

As we age there is usually a change in our gut and/or digestive process. Ideally, we all need to slow down and chew our food, so that it can mix evenly with our saliva. This precious saliva allows the nutrients to travel smoothly down the esophagus and into our stomachs. By slowing down and chewing our food, we may also lessen the chances of choking. If our food is mixed well with hydrochloric acid in the stomach, it will increase the absorption of nutrients. Food is then free to travel through the small intestine and on into the large intestine with the help of the liver, pancreas, and gall bladder. We can help this process by adding fresh produce and water to our everyday consumption.

There is an interesting gut/brain connection that creates an internal feedback loop. Many of us have experienced a case of nervousness (butterflies) in our stomach before an important presentation, meeting, or possible confrontation. The gastrointestinal tract is extremely sensitive to emotion, which is why feelings (our own and others) such as danger, fear, anxiety, sadness, elation, anger, etc., can trigger a *"gut reaction."* In other words, the brain has a direct effect on the stomach, and vice versa. This internal stress may sometimes result in gastrointestinal conditions such as bloating, cramps, constipation, diarrhea, excess gas, heartburn, irritable bowel syndrome, gastric reflux, nausea, stomachaches, and ulcers.

The best way to think about this connection is to imagine that there is a highway of nerves between the brain and the digestive system; and that messages can flow in two directions. In fact, ninety-five percent of the body's serotonin, the hormone that helps control mood, is found in the digestive system, not the brain. So, when the gut is happy, we are happy! And on the flip side, when the brain is stressed, it sends a cascade of hormones that can turn the stomach upside down. In a panic we freeze, flee, or stuff our face with more food or drink to calm and sooth our jangled nerves.

Most of us eat too fast. Your challenge in the next few weeks is to see if you can slow down your need to eat quickly. Can you put your eating utensils down between each bite? Does an electronic device, book, newspaper, or person distract you from tasting, chewing, and swallowing your food?

Notice whether adding more pauses between each bite of food and sip of liquid can improve your digestion. This practice may give you more of a feeling of satiation at the end of your meal.

4. Moving Assets:
Spring Cleaning Year Around

The conventional asset list may include real estate, cars, recreational vehicles or cabins, clothes, furniture, paintings, stocks, jewelry, collections, family heirlooms, or anything a person has decided has personal value. Then there are those hard-to-see assets or what I like to call *invisible assets*. How does one put a cash value on friends, family, relationships, education, music, nature, and love? I highly recommend that you begin to literally take inventory of your visible and invisible assets.

Before you hit the panic button, hear me out. Think of physics; everything has energy. Most of us could use a little more energy in our lives, and I am going to show you the fastest calorie-free path to lightening up, and adding more peace and less stress to the last few chapters of your life. If this seems daunting or overwhelming, I want you to take a deep breath and take the next few weeks to question absolutely everything you touch and the people you interact with. Ask yourself:

a) *If my home burned down today, would I really miss this item? Does this item give me joy?*

b) *If this person simply disappeared today would I miss them?* If yes, please let them know right now how much you treasure your relationship.

I am NOT suggesting getting rid of every possession or every annoying person in your life. I am just asking you to mindfully *re-purpose* or *re-allocate* your physical possessions before you die. I am also asking you to realize that with our limited time on earth you may not want to spend hours of your precious time on a person or activity that drains your energy. The hardest part of this whole process is to start! Your first assignment is to stop reading RIGHT NOW and go find something small in your living space that you would like to give away. Place it in a labeled box or bag. Tomorrow know that you will add one thing a day for the next thirty days. And then donate the entire box or bag to an organization of your choice.

NOTE: *If you live with other people this assignment may be difficult, especially if your significant other is very attached to his/her things. The best action here is to only deal with anything that is yours. Unless you are moving right away, there is no reason to let go of your couches, recliners, dining room table, bed, dressers, etc. However, you can clear the clutter around these things so that they can breathe and fully serve their purpose. It's also helpful to do your research now: decide and write down ideas of where all those big items will go if you are suddenly looking at long-term care, hospice, and death. Most important, please do not give away that recliner because you dislike it and your partner absolutely loves it. This may be a good time to ask your significant other about where they think all of your mutual possessions should go when you no longer can take care of them. They may surprise you with their answer.*

Please remember that all these changes work best when they come from love. Start with changing yourself; your actions may trigger your family and friends to follow your example. If you are dealing with the fact that your spouse, significant other, or children are resistant to the idea that you will eventually die, it is YOUR responsibility to broach the subject. If the resistance is thick and heavy, then you will have more challenges; however, do not give up. They will eventually see the wisdom of your actions.

The best legacy we can leave our loved ones is with memories of our actions, including having difficult conversations. Be sure to always be polite and aware of others' space: *I've been thinking about what is going to happen to everything in this house when I can no longer take care of things. When is a good time for us to talk about it?* Most people appreciate the courtesy of being asked, and not told. You may even find that they have been thinking about the same issue, but were hesitant to broach the topic for whatever reason. Do yourself a favor and START THE CONVERSATION.

If you are facing a mega-house of full inventory, you may choose to start placing stickers discreetly on all your possessions, and writing down who will receive them when you die. If you think there may be a problem, just take photos and label them. Make sure your attorney or trusted loved ones have copies. Or you may want to give these items to their recipients today. They may also choose to decline an item simply because it doesn't work for them right now; see if they can find a storage place and/or new home for that item. Be sure to remember that the recipient may not want that chair, painting, or piece of jewelry.

This is an opportunity to keep all doors open. Ask the recipient if you can give the item to someone else. Most people appreciate the gesture, but not everyone is interested in our heirlooms.

NOTE: *It is NOT your responsibility to take care of your heirlooms for your heirs, unless you choose to be a storage unit.*

I know that internal bodily cleanses are quite popular; however, I highly recommend starting with an external cleanse. How much stuff do we really need and want? I know several seniors who had emotional meltdowns as they downsized – from their overstuffed three-bedroom homes with an overflowing two-car garage, basement, attic, and storage units – into a studio apartment. Some individuals may also have to deal with selling a boat, second home, or big-ticket toys that they hadn't used in years. If you are using these items less and less, and you are certainly getting older every day, why not start lightening up today? It will not only save you a ton of stress, but when the time comes it will be easier to gracefully slide into that one-bedroom apartment, studio or assisted living center. Eventually you will be leaving all these assets so why not practice releasing them now and saving your heirs a ton of work?

You may choose to take everything out of every closet, shelf, and storage area of your home. Or you may start with one drawer at a time. You know yourself, you may even try an experiment. If you tend to be very cautious and maybe even indecisive, you may want to move things to a designated closet or the garage, and let them bench cool for a month.

Just don't wait too long; that defeats the purpose of moving things out. This also works if you tend to move too fast and sometimes regret your decisions. You may choose to pick one day each week to work on one area of your home or one group of items: shoes, books, clothes, closets, kitchen shelves, files, etc. Either way, find a system that works for you and start moving.

And those annoying people whom you would like to get out of your life? This is not as easy as dropping off a chair at Goodwill. However, you can learn to navigate around difficult people, including your family and friends. Everyone has a gift. Your job is to focus on the good and gracefully avoid situations that cause you lasting stress. Being a wise sage is looking at the minefields and avoiding them as much as possible. This includes finding exit doors that do not cause further harm to your loved ones, including yourself.

NOTE: *Many of us may be in a relationship, partnership, or marriage where our partner is not interested in any or all of the above. Your challenge is to continue on your mission and hopefully, by your example, be able to communicate the importance of taking care of the business of living. We are not here to bully or shame people about their behavior; we are here to lead ourselves and our loved ones into living a lighter, juicier, and happier life.*

Food for Thought: Researching Your Options Before A Crisis

There are many community programs that will assist seniors living in their home for as long as possible. Some of these programs even provide personal services such as bathing and prescription compliance, however you may not be ready for that level of care. So get creative and start brainstorming your options. Possibilities may include renting a bedroom/bathroom or part of your home to a college student, a single working person, or a young family in exchange for home maintenance, yard work, and running errands. Start your research now and discuss options with your loved ones so that you do not have to start with an unexpected emergency. And if a crisis does occur, as in a sudden injury and/or surgery, you will have several plans and options already lined up.

5. Practicing Stillness:
Doing Nothing

Have you ever sat quietly watching clouds in the sky, a setting sun, or a rising moon? Practicing stillness is an art and a science that is accessible to all of us; it is invaluable to cultivating peacefulness in all aspects of our life. Being in stillness is often called meditation; however, that sometimes conjures up sitting on the floor with your legs crossed, staring into a candle and chanting. The truth is that meditation and practicing stillness come in many different flavors. Experiment and be open to just sitting and staring out the window. Just sit and breathe.

Whenever you are feeling unbalanced, upset, or even just bored, see if you can shift your focus with a mini-meditation. Do you have a favorite prayer, song, mantra, or poem that gives you a feeling of peace and quiet? Or you may choose to take a few deep breaths. It is so easy to get caught up with all the *lions, tigers, and bears* that may (or may not) be out to get you. Or maybe some tasks belong to someone else and you are taking them on as your pet projects. As one of my friends likes to remind me: *Be careful who or what you feed.*

It takes discipline not to get swept away in the current of nonstop news, emails, and electronic updates. It's OK to feel overwhelmed as we get sucked into a media or family hurricane/tornado. Our challenge is to find that *stillness in the eye of the storm.*

Can we train ourselves to pause before responding? Even if your stillness only lasts a few breaths, it is a priceless tool for practicing meditation for the rest of your life.

One of the best meditation rooms I know is the bathroom, specifically the bathtub. Just sit in a warm bubble bath and do absolutely nothing. Bathtubs offer a perfect meditation container with the added benefit of emerging with a clean body. I do know that some people prefer showers; however I find that it is healthy to mix it up. You may even want to try a flotation tank; the new tanks have soft lights and you can leave the lid open. Check out your local spa scene. They are usually listed as "flotation therapy." Most people report a feeling of deep relaxation and meditative state, regardless of their age.

There is no magic recipe or meditation pill that will give you serenity throughout the day. It is up to you to find your own techniques for recharging your batteries. Remember that doing nothing *is* something.

Food for Thought

"Walking is man's best medicine."

— Hippocrates

"If you are in a bad mood, go for a walk.
If you are still in a bad mood, go for another walk."

— Hippocrates

ELEMENT FIVE

Rest & Relaxation: The Icing on the Cake

Years ago, when I was working for the Arthritis Foundation as a health educator, the primary message was that arthritis was not a death sentence; it was a call to action. It was an opportunity to modify one's lifestyle. Individuals were encouraged to listen closely to their body and take "rest" breaks between activities. This philosophy applied to everything from exercise, chores, activities, medications, working, and socializing. In fact, their whole philosophy made so much sense to me that it has stayed with me all these years. Most of us know when we have done too much and sense when we have not done enough. The key is to find a balance and as in *Goldilocks and The Three Bears* – not too much and not too little!

Rest and relaxation are two different words but I am going to combine them. My definition of rest and relaxation is any activity that gives you pleasure and makes you feel good while being legal, ethical, and not causing harm to any person, place, or thing. The definition of rest and relaxation is very personal. Although we usually equate rest and relaxation as a passive activity, it can also be incredibly active.

Gardening may relax you, but it stresses me out. Baking cakes may be your stress releaser, but I'd rather chop vegetables. Running marathons or a 10K may make you happy, but it's not on my list. The bottom line is that we all need to respect an individual's activity choices and take responsibility for the activities that work for us today. We also need to be flexible. We may no longer be able to run, ski, and jog, however maybe we can walk, snowshoe, and swim.

One of the most popular yoga postures done at the end of a yoga class is called *Savasana* – the corpse pose. The ancient yogis recommended this practice as a reminder to all of us that we are all going to eventually leave our physical body on earth. Since death and dying are such loaded words in our culture, modern day yoga teachers and practitioners will often refer to this final resting posture as *The Relaxation Pose.*

This posture is a wonderful opportunity to remind us to take a break, let go, and sink into the earth. It is also a reminder that we are constantly surrounded by death and dying. Everything around us is always changing: from the flowers in the vase on our table, to our bodies, our relationships, and even the fresh food in our refrigerator which will eventually decompose. We need to take these everyday opportunities to realize just how very precious this moment is, that our lives here on earth are incredibly short, and that we can die at any moment.

Most people whom I have discussed death and dying with agree that they would like to die as peacefully as possible, preferably at home in their own beds. It is up to us to create the opportunity to have our final wishes supported. We also need to be cognizant of the reality that we may die in a facility or away from home. It is up to us to change the culture of talking about the reality of our death and dying with our friends, family, and medical practitioners.

The most important words your loved ones will want to hear from you, preferably before you die, are "*I love you.*" When I was working as a grief counselor I can tell you that the survivors who heard their dying loved one say those three words simply grieved differently. They knew that despite any issues they were truly loved.

Take a few minutes and look at what is really important to you. *What would happen if you died in the next five minutes?* It may be impossible to die with a clean desk, bills paid, all the laundry done, no dishes in the sink, thank you notes written, phone calls completed, and all relationship rifts healed. However, this idea of dying could also be taken as a wakeup call to action, to work on your lists of unfinished tasks, projects, and even your bucket list! It may even entail making an appointment with your attorney, calling a loved one, writing a love letter or dropping off a load of household items to a thrift store, women's shelter, or recycling center. In fact, stop reading right now and go do one thing on your list – it may be a phone call – but do it now. I guarantee you will feel better!

Our responsibility is to make room for completing these tasks and finding more pleasurable opportunities in our lives today. There is nothing wrong with creating more loving, fun, and lighter moments in your life right now. Put that list of *things to do* right where you can see it, and choose to tackle it with humor, grace, and tenacity over the next few weeks.

Food for Thought

The ancient yogis recommended taking deep,

mindful breaths throughout the day as a reminder

that we are all going to leave our physical body. We

need to realize just how precious our breath is, and

that our lives here on earth are incredibly short.

Activity: Breathe

If you are not in a situation that requires your full attention, such as driving a car, slicing a bagel or operating equipment, the following three movements are great transitions to do before going on to your next activity.

1. Close your eyes and take three of the deepest *inhale-pause-exhale-pause* breaths that you have taken all day. When you are finished, open your eyes slowly and savor the quiet, before you move on to your next activity.

2. See if you can inhale and squeeze your fingers on each hand into a very tight fist. Pause and then exhale, splaying open your fingers as widely as they will go. Feel free to do this several times before you move on to your next activity.

3. Jump up and down three times. If your knees or hips are too vulnerable, just shake your body from head to toe without lifting your feet off the ground. Even standing in one place and wiggling will induce a giggle, and maybe even a smile!

Yoga Rx: Rest & Relaxation

1. **Favorite Activities: Rediscovering & Learning Something New**

2. **Curiosity: Expanding Your Universe**

3. **Sleep: A Precious Vitamin**

4. **Transitioning into the Final Phase of Your life**

5. **Practice Dying: Letting Go One Day at a Time**

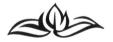

1. Favorite Activities:
Rediscovering & Learning Something New

Regular physical activity can boost energy, reduce stress, and even help you sleep better at night. Many of us experience various levels of physical discomfort throughout the day so listen closely to your body. It is helpful to think of what you enjoyed doing as a child. Maybe you loved climbing trees, bicycling, and swimming. Get creative and find a safe walking path with trees, ride a stationary bike, or check out your local swimming pools.

Ask your friends what they are doing. Maybe you will get invited to a Zumba, Tai Chi, Qi Gong, or weight lifting class. And remember to walk as much as possible. Even if you only take a walk around your apartment, home, or living center – keep walking. If your knees and hips are pain free, walking up and down stairs is always a plus.

You may also want to consult your health care practitioner or a physical therapist to create a workout plan that's right for you. You may be surprised at how much you can do without leaving your home. Whatever you do, always listen to your body, and make sure you can always breathe comfortably.

- Take a moment to make a list of every activity that you like to do and every activity that you would like to try before you die. Find a way to bring those activities into your life today. You may no longer be physically up to a ten-mile hike; however, you may be able to find shorter trails and local walkways. See how creative you can be in trying the activities on your list.

You may also enjoy living vicariously through books, magazines, and movies. Most libraries have *free* tables where you can pick up interesting magazines on travel, fishing, bicycling, cooking, and design. Think of all these activities as brain enhancers, lighting up your synapses and expanding your universe.

- Be curious. Check out activity options at senior citizen centers, gyms, YMCA/YWCA, and public libraries. Find a friend to go with you and/or start your own activity circle; invite a friend or friends to your home to watch a movie, share a meal, or enjoy a walk together.

- Walking around an indoor shopping mall or up and down the aisles of a big store can also give you an opportunity to get out and about – and offer you a great opportunity to LOOK, but not BUY. (Even if it's 70% off, walk out without purchasing anything and you will be 100% ahead!) If you are more homebound, don't be discouraged. Look around your living space and find opportunities to move, stretch, and bend throughout the day.

- As one of my friends pointed out, it is good to find another heartbeat to connect with every day. This heartbeat can be in the form of a dog, cat, smiling barista, walking buddy, exercise friend, favorite nurse, massage therapist, or librarian. The smiles connected to the heart are priceless and it can make all the difference in adding pleasure to our lives.

- Whatever you do, remember to always listen to your body and make sure you are breathing comfortably. If you do get winded, stressed, or feel pressure of any kind, simply stop and recalibrate. See if you can identify what really is going on. Be curious and brutally honest with yourself. Give yourself the gift of compassion. Your body, mind, and spirit will thank you.

2. Curiosity: Expanding Your Universe

Curiosity is the desire to explore, to learn, and to get to know someone or something. It involves a spirit of inquisitiveness and the ability to ask *WHY*. What happened to that curious funny three-year-old we once were? That child who got excited about sunbeams, flying squirrels, and a slug on the front walkway? Where did s/he go?

One of the "youngest" elders I have ever met was my father's cousin Fran. She had lived through the depression, World War II, multiple family traumas including the early death of her spouse, and yet she was always asking: *Why? What do YOU think? If you could change the situation, what would you do?* Once I asked her what she thought about our current president and she said: *I already know what I think, it's much more interesting to find out what you think, because then I may just have to change my mind!*

The juiciest seniors I know are the ones who keep exploring. They are always reading a new book, going to lectures, listening to books on tape, meeting new people, taking classes, and going on mini-trips. And just because you take a class, does not mean that you must become a gourmet chef, open a gallery, or publish a book. It's all about keeping your brain cells juicy and keeping your social skills active.

Please do not think that you must spend a lot of money to do something new. Libraries, schools, community centers, bookstores, movie theaters, galleries, and museums all offer free and/or senior discounts to many wonderful activities.

By the way, do not hesitate to go by yourself. I guarantee if you go with an open heart, with absolutely no expectations, you will find yourself smiling and sitting down next to someone, and making a new friend. It's also good to just get comfortable going solo. I love going to the movies and traveling by myself. You will be surprised how much more you see when you are not distracted by talking or being with another person. And better yet, if you are not your own best friend, who is?

3. *Sleep: A Precious Vitamin*

Most of us have had the unfortunate experience of not getting enough sleep. And as we all know, sleep is a very personal issue, and yet the controversy continues as to how much sleep we need to successfully function. Sleep is technically the suspension of voluntary bodily functions, usually marked by complete or partial consciousness – in other words, not being awake.

Sleeping well gives the body/mind a chance to refresh itself. There is also evidence that when we sleep, the brain performs a self-cleaning or "reboot" process. Sleep allows the body to repair cell damage and invigorate the immune system. Our brains, bones, skin, organs, and muscles need to rest and rejuvenate. This can explain why after a deep sleep, we wake refreshed; and why after a night of constantly waking up to go to the bathroom, ruminating over an issue, or listening to the loud music next door, we do not function well the following day. Recent studies have also linked insufficient sleep with an increased risk of breast cancer in women, diabetes, obesity, and cardiovascular diseases. I am not saying that insufficient sleep will cause cancer; it is just one of the many factors that affect your overall health profile. The science has already proved that with sufficient sleep, we are able to make healthier decisions, enjoy our life more, and usually live longer.

Sleep was so important to the ancient yogis that they developed a practice called *Yoga Nidra / Yoga Sleep*. This is a form of relaxation that can best be described as a *state of mind between being awake and being in a deep sleep.* Deep sleep means that someone must shake you to get you up or you need an alarm clock. In *Yoga Sleep* the body looks like it is sleeping, but the mind is functioning at a deeper level. If someone yelled "fire" you would definitely respond immediately.

I like to practice deep relaxation before I go to sleep at night. This ritual especially works if I have insomnia, am angry about something that happened during the day, or am worried about a future event. When I explained it to a dear friend of mine, she laughed and said: *Oh, that's what we call meditation.* Another friend calls it her *evening gratitude list.* I simply call it *deep relaxation* or *my organic sleeping pill.* I sincerely hope that you take my basic *Yoga Sleep* outline and experiment, adapt, or modify it to fit your needs. Be aware that every time you practice this it will be different, and if you are unattached to how it should look and feel, you will truly be practicing your very own version of *Yoga Sleep.*

My Version of Yoga Sleep

1. Begin by preparing your body for sleep. When you create consistent bedtime rituals, the body/mind can begin to relax knowing what is coming next. I like to wash my face, brush and floss my teeth. If I am cold I like to put lotion on my feet, and then put on a pair of socks to keep my feet warm.

2. Make sure your bedroom is as neat and organized as possible. This may include closing closet doors, hanging up clothes, and making sure all electronics

are off. This includes hiding all LED light screens – especially phones, tablets, and digital clocks by the bedside.

3. If you have bedroom curtains or blinds that do not completely block out the light, you may want to install heavy duty blackout curtains. They not only block outside light, but can serve as a sound buffer. You may also want to try an eye mask.

4. Remember that everyone has their own personal temperature zone for sleeping, which sometimes makes it difficult to sleep with someone who has a different preference. It may take some experimentation before you and your partner find the best combination of chill, heat, blanket thickness, and cat/dogs/children in bed. Remember that environments including people may change, so it is up to you to take responsibility for your comfort, safety, and well-being.

5. Clean sheets, blankets, and pillows often help to create a comfortable nest and are important in creating the opportunity for a restful sleep. Some people like to put a pillow under their knees or use an eye pillow to relax their eyes. Experiment and do what works for you, knowing that you may make modifications at any time.

6. I find that the most comfortable position to start in is lying on my back and doing a body scan, starting with my toes and moving up to the crown of my head. I simply name each body part and ask it to "relax" and

"let go." The image of melting into the mattress also works for me.

7. Sometimes I put my hands on my belly as I lengthen my inhales, pauses, and exhales. There is something relaxing about feeling the belly rise and fall with each inhale and each exhale. I simply silently say: *Inhale belly raises, pause, exhale belly falls, pause, inhale …*

8. After a few rounds of breathing I may choose to leave my hands on my belly, place them at my heart center between my breasts, or leave my arms by my side with my palms facing up. Then I start my gratitude list. Sometimes nothing comes to mind so I will start with thanking my firm mattress, warm quilt, and full belly. If nothing comes to mind I will go through the house in my mind thanking everything that I have including running water, fresh towels, electricity, books, food in the fridge. Sometimes, after mentally walking through my home I will walk out the front door and out into the neighborhood, through my favorite parks… the journey of gratitude is endless.

   Sometimes an unpleasant stressor may pop up unexpectedly; usually I try to not ignore it and breathe into it. If it is something that I need to remember to do I simply stop and write it down. Yes, I keep a pad of paper by my bed and have been known to write down an errand, key words to a dream, or an idea. Once it is written, I can get back to relaxing. In this state of relaxation, I can often conjure up compassion for myself and the other person or situation that is causing me grief. If I feel any tension, I can bless the situation and tell myself I will deal with it tomorrow. Sometimes I take my mind to the beach, and just sit watching the waves go in and out. Or I take myself on a beautiful mountain trail or visualize myself doing yoga postures. It's good to have a list of options to go through, including counting sheep jumping over a fence. One of my friends puts herself to sleep by playing the alphabet game: *A is for apple, B is for boy.* She says she never makes it to Z! And if you really want a challenge, try doing the alphabet backwards!

I encourage you to experiment and personalize the above steps towards creating a restful sleep. Some of my friends and family use a mantra, music, or a favorite prayer to ease them into sleep. There are many excellent relaxation practices available on CDs or podcasts. There are also white noise machines. Ask your friends if they have any sleeping tips; it's a great conversation starter! And if you want to get really scientific, keep a sleep journal and see if you can figure out the elements that go into getting a good night's sleep. The answers may surprise you.

4. Transitioning into the Final Phase of Your Life

The first time I read about the Hindu tradition of the *Four Ashramas of Life* I thought it was rather archaic and simplistic. But now that I am approaching my twilight years I can see that the ancients may have been on to something. They claimed that the ideal life span was eighty-four years plus, with each of the four stages divided into roughly twenty-one years. The goal was to take responsibility for each stage of your life so that you would be free to literally wander off into the sunset during your final years. The stages have since been extended into twenty-five years per phase and it goes something like this:

Age 0 to 21 or 0 to 25:   In youth, the student learns and studies everything they can about life. This is a time of exploration, training, discipline, and finding one's place in the family and community. There is an emphasis on taking responsibility for your physical and academic gifts. It also includes demonstrating respect for your elders and honoring their guidance. This is generally referred to as the *Student Phase.*

Ages 22 to 42 or 26 to 50:   This is called the *Householder Phase*, when one lives with a spouse, children, and possibly an extended family of parents, in-laws, siblings, and cousins. One does not necessarily have to be married or have children; one's career, passion for art or politics and/or travel can be your "child." It is all about nurturing others through one's activities, interests, and duties. In this phase, community is very important, whether it be through work, church, or any organization that you choose to support with your time, energy, and money.

Ages 43 to 63 or 51 to 75:   As one's children, projects and activities grow up, move on or shift, the householder is encouraged to mentor others and start to expand their own personal spiritual practice. This is often referred to as the *Retirement Phase*. Many people begin to "downsize" their activities, possessions and work life. They may choose to travel, give possessions and responsibilities to others, and move towards a less busy lifestyle.

Ages 64 to 84 or 76 to 100+:   In this final stage, you are given permission to let go of all responsibilities and let your family and society support you. It is sometimes referred to the *Renunciation Phase*. There are no longer any professional, social, political obligations, or chores that you need to do. *You are free to literally walk off into the sunset.* You have earned your *Wise Elder Badge!*

As my friend Bill says: *That means I can finally sit on my front porch in my underwear.* He is of course referring to his cottage in the woods.

On a more serious note, there is sometimes quite a bit of confusion and fear surrounding this phase. It sometimes coincides with retirement and the awkwardness of meeting someone, shaking hands and no longer being employed as an accountant, teacher, or nurse. *Hi, I am Margaret and I am a* _____? We are now free to figure out who we are, so that we can greet others with openness and not be burdened with a label. Even the word "retirement" is loaded. This is the time to seriously look at what we do all day and figure out a graceful way to connect with people without the burden of a label.

Please remember that none of these four stages are set in stone. Most of us will not fit neatly into four little boxes. Like the four seasons of the year, there may be transitional periods, as in being semi-retired. The truth is that everyone has a different life path to fulfill.

The task here is to raise your awareness of where you are in your life and to look honestly at where you want to be before you die. Some personalities need to be constantly surrounded by lots of activity, whereas others crave so much time alone that their caregivers often panic. It is our responsibility to find our own level of socialization and be fully aware of our changes as we move into our final stage. It is also important to always communicate our needs and wants with the people we love, including ourselves. We are the pioneers charting new courses and opportunities. If we do not share our process, the next generation will not benefit from our stories and wisdom.

I hope this gives you some inspiration to use the above four stages to map out your life to date. Making a time line may help you focus on where you would like to go or what you would like to do in your final stage. Be curious about what comes up for you. Remember that everyone will have a different time line and not everything is set in stone.

5. Practice Dying:
Letting Go One Day at A Time

Years ago, I did a death and dying exercise during our hospice volunteer training that I will never forget. We were each given ten index cards and asked to write down ten people, activities, or things that were close to our heart – in other words our top ten loves. When we were all finished writing, our leader asked us to look closely at all our cards. We then had to choose to give up one card and put it in a basket that was sitting in the middle of the table. She slowly asked us to give up one card at a time, until we were sitting holding on to our last card. By then most of us were crying, realizing just how hard it is going to be to let go of everything we love when we die. The last card was the hardest – it was the love of our life – the person or animal we loved the most and had to say goodbye to. Yes, it was "just an exercise," but it was also a wake-up call to treasure those moments, because ultimately all the cards will be collected. (Detailed instructions for this exercise are in the Appendix.)

Death and dying are often difficult topics to discuss, simply because we don't know exactly when we are going to die or even the circumstances that will lead up to our death. The list of possibilities and variables makes for a very complicated algorithm which would probably challenge the most sophisticated programmer. Yes, I am sure you read about Oscar the cat, who could predict when a patient was about to die. He lived in a nursing home and would sniff the air and often curl up on the bed next to a patient. The nursing staff quickly learned when to call the patient's family to come and say goodbye. And sure enough, each one of them died shortly after Oscar's visit. And yes, there are studies that can predict your death if you are terminally ill in palliative care; however, we all know someone who lived longer than expected.

It's hard to imagine physically exiting our bodies and literally not being HERE! I am not going to delve into the existence of God, a higher power, souls, reincarnation, or the afterlife. Those are very personal topics and unique to everyone. However, I do think we owe it to ourselves and our loved ones to start to deal with the reality of our own death and dying.

The good news is that it is not necessarily depressing to do this homework; in fact, most people find it liberating. Remember that clearing the clutter from your life includes not only physical possessions but also people and obligations that no longer have value or meaning to you. If the following list of ideas seems daunting, just do a little bit every day and I promise that you will feel more optimistic, lighter, and even joyful.

a) **There are many philosophies** on how to declutter your physical possessions. The ultimate litmus test is: If a fire destroyed your entire living space (yes, including that storage unit), would you really miss this item? Would you replace it? Most of us know we can always get another mattress, couch, car, towels, dishes, etc. and we can always tell the story about that wonderful item – but it is replaceable. So, do your heirs a favor today and ask them if they want anything; better yet, give it to them right now. And if they say *No thank you,* honor their wishes. Your task is to find good homes for everything except the necessities. Bonus points: Less housework!

b) **The most important aspect** of finding homes for all your things is to NOT add more clutter into your physical space. Do you really NEED another storage bin? A bowl? A painting? If someone has given you a book, a piece of clothing, or a vase, ask them if they want it back. Is it OK to pass it along to someone else? Encourage people to ask for permission before they give, re-gift, or dump stuff on you. Be sure to extend this courtesy to others, so that you are not sending a box of books to someone who couldn't care less about your "gift." Find good homes for your stuff. Your living space will thank you.

c) **We are not perfect.** In fact, most of us have hurt someone we have loved. This lack if communication is often referred to as "unfinished business." It is important to remember that the other person may not even be aware of your issue, but if the regret is still sitting in your heart, you may want to resolve it before you die. If this task feels impossible to do, you may ease into it by simply writing a letter of apology to everyone on your list. It doesn't have to be long and you don't necessarily have to send it. In fact the person may be dead. You are simply clearing the slate, washing your internal windows. I can't begin to tell you how liberating it is to say: "*I am so sorry I hurt you, please forgive me.*" Remember, they may not forgive you, and that is their choice. As hard as it may be, let it go.

d) **Write your obituary.** This is an interesting exercise because it will help you focus on your legacy. How do you want your life to read? Would someone who knows you well agree with what you say? Would a perfect stranger reading your story have a sense of your values, ethics, and priorities? If this feels like a daunting task, just look at next Sunday's obituaries and copy a template of an obituary that resonates with you. Substitute yourself, your family, activities, and passions into a story written in the third person. You may even want to write an epitaph for your gravestone, even if you are cremated. What sound bite would you like to leave behind? What song or poem really reflects who you are? Be sure to include these documents with your important papers.

e) **Documents.** Always keep your loved one informed of where your written final wishes are located. This includes important documents such as advanced directives, wills, and trusts. Better yet, on an annual basis make sure your caregivers know and understand exactly what you want concerning life support, organ donations, and burial/cremation. It is a good idea to give updated copies of all important written paperwork, signed and dated, to your family, friends, and health practitioners. Not everyone will be able to support you, but even if they don't agree with you, it will help them do their own homework, and hopefully open the door to more dialog and conversations. The best times to update your documents are at the first of the new year, on your birthday, or at the end of the year. Some people choose to update their families and friends on April 15 with a sense of humor about death and taxes.

NOTE: *If you are in hospice care, their care team will review your advanced healthcare directives with you. If you are in pre-hospice or dealing with a chronic condition, you may want to have a packet of all your current documents within easy reach. You may choose to keep this packet near the front door, so that your caregivers can grab it and be ready to respond in case of a medical crisis. Or you may choose to keep your information on a thumb drive or the cloud where it is easily accessible.*

If you are experiencing a medical emergency or crisis, I highly recommend that you keep a blank notebook with your packet so that you or your caregivers can write down the names of the people you interact with, their recommendations, along with the date and time. It will also provide a priceless backup in the midst of information overload, avoiding possible medication mix-ups, and remembering which health care worker suggested what procedure.

Your caregiver can also take photos on their cell phone, of medications, medical personnel face/name, and any other information that may get lost in the shuffle of a crisis.

Rx: *Practice Leaving Your Body*

There is a wonderful posture that is usually done at the end of every yoga class called *Savasana* or *Shavasana*. The literal translation is "corpse pose," but most people refer to it as the "relaxation posture." It is usually done lying on your back with your arms and legs relaxed at your side and your eyes closed. You may choose to place a bolster under your knees to take any pressure off your lower back, add a blanket for additional warmth, or place a soft towel or eye pillow over your eyes to further relax your eyes and face.

The purpose of *Savasana* is to rejuvenate the body, mind, and spirit. It is all about giving the body a chance to recharge its batteries. Yoga students are encouraged to *melt into the floor* and *let it all go.* My own experience as a yoga student and teacher is that this is usually the most popular and most treasured posture of an entire practice. Yes, you may fall asleep, or have a cosmic insight, or update that task list, or maybe just listen to the sounds around you. Or as one of my yoga buddies likes to remind me: where else can adults lie down on the floor in the middle of the day and it is socially acceptable!

HOMEWORK: If you can, right now I want you to go lie down on the floor, your couch, recliner or bed, and just let everything go. If you can't quite get into it, just take a deep inhale and squeeze your body as tightly as you can and then slowly exhale. Let yourself melt like an ice cube on a scorching hot summer day. Let everything melt into the earth. Give yourself a few minutes of doing absolutely nothing and see what happens.

Food for Thought

One of the joys of yoga is when all five elements:

Breathing, Internal Lifts, Gazing In & Out,

Movement and Rest & Relaxation

are all working together.

Usually we are so happy, relaxed, and peaceful

we don't even realize that we are

doing or experiencing yoga!

A New Perspective: From This Day Forward

Throughout history there has been a constant search for the secret to longevity, happiness, and love. Most of us yearn for some version of *Shangri-La*: a peaceful place with no pain, suffering, or conflicts of any kind. However, the reality is that no such place exists and we are stuck in the daily grind of keeping all the balls in the air. The good news is that these yoga tools give us an opportunity to create instant islands of calm wherever we are in our life. They are timeless, ageless, and can be practiced until the day we die.

One of the best tools I have found to create a little bliss in the moment is simply *Walking Tall*. Please note that the following instructions can also be adapted to *Sitting Tall* or *Lying Down Tall*.

Rx: Walking Tall

The next time you get up out of your chair or are walking from one area to another, notice your posture and what you are thinking. Many of us are so focused on getting to the next task that we are not even aware of our body moving through space. We may be juggling multiple tasks, errands, and conversations in our head that when we walk into the kitchen we may not even remember what we are looking for.

Or maybe you are walking with a friend and you are so busy thinking of what you are going to say next that you trip on a rock on the trail. Notice what happens when you are trying to text, walk, and think all at the same time.

No wonder we are often exhausted, distracted, and frustrated. We are trying to listen to several radio stations simultaneously instead of just doing one thing at a time. The following sequence is a great way to lift your body, mind, and spirit. It will also increase your focus, balance, and serenity.

1. STOP. FREEZE. LOOK down at your feet and notice if your body weight is equality distributed between your two feet. Are you leaning more to one side than the other? Inhale and see if you can lift your toes up towards your face. Even if you have shoes on, can you do a little stretch? Then as you exhale, slowly release your toes to the ground. Feel your feet pressing down evenly into the floor. See if you can rock side to side, back and forth, heel to toe. Notice your balance. When you feel balanced with your feet firmly on the ground, inhale, squeeze your thighs, and feel your

kneecaps lifting. As slowly as you can on the next exhale, release, and soften your thighs.

NOTE: *If you have any knee issues, including artificial knees, please check with a licensed practitioner before doing this knee lift or anything involving your knee joints.*

2. Next, put your hand on your belly button. Inhale as you pull your belly button towards your spine. This is a very subtle internal lift so you may not see it but you will feel it. After some practice you will be able to do this without your hand on your belly. As you inhale, feel your stomach muscles lifting the diaphragm, and the "sit bones" dropping. (The anatomy term is the *ischial tuberosity.* These sitting bones are protected by the *gluteus maximus.*) This gentle tilt protects the lower back and strengthens your core muscles.

NOTE: *If you have recently had any abdominal issues or surgery, or are pregnant, please skip the above section.*

3. Bring your attention to your shoulders and see if you can inhale as you lift your shoulders up to your ears and squeeze. As you exhale release your shoulders down and away from your ears. It usually takes me several squeezes before I feel any release. Sometimes I like to add some shoulder rolls, using my breath to lift my shoulders up to my ears, forward, down and back around. I like to do a few rounds of rolling my shoulders backwards and forwards, clockwise and counterclockwise. Some individuals also find relief by taking a deep inhale and then on the exhale dropping their right ear to their right shoulder; and

then inhaling back up, pausing in the center, and then exhaling left ear towards the left shoulder. I sometimes like to hold this posture for several breaths – just inhaling, pausing, and exhaling to release any neck tension. You may also get some relief by exhaling as you drop your chin to your chest, pausing, and then on an inhale lifting your chin back to center. I highly recommend trying a few of these variations to find a stretch that works for you.

NOTE: *If you have any injuries or traumas to the neck and shoulders, please be very gentle and consult with a health care provider before aggravating or causing more discomfort and harm.*

4. Next, take a deep inhale and exhale, then continue breathing as you feel me standing behind you gently pulling your hair up from the crown of your head, and elongating your spine so that you are just a bit taller.

NOTE: *If you are bald, then imagine that you have a full head of hair and feel the top of your skull lifting up to touch the ceiling.*

Do a quick scan from the crown of your head through your body and down to your toes. See if you can send your breath up and down your body – toes to head and head to toes. Always make sure that your face is soft, your jaw is unclenched, and your shoulders are down and away from your ears. Feel your body totally aligned as you walk forward breathing evenly, feeling stronger, more focused, and yet relaxed.

Walking Tall may sound complicated; however, it is a great yoga practice that will give you a lifetime of benefits. The more you practice, the easier it will become, until it is second nature. Throughout your day, look for opportunities for *Walking Tall*. When you get out of bed in the morning see if you can *Walk Tall* to the bathroom, then to the kitchen, and then from room to room, and on out into your busy day. *Walking Tall* is a great mini-meditation, especially when you add your mindful inhales, pauses, and exhales. You will find yourself arriving at your destination refreshed and carrying less tension. It will add a bit of bounce to your step and may even put a smile on your face.

Walking Tall may also be practiced while sitting or lying down. If you are sitting in a chair, you can still wiggle your toes, squeeze your thighs, pull your belly button towards your spine, roll your shoulders up and around, drop the chin to your chest and look up with a smile as you balance your head evenly on the top of your spine.

The action of pushing the top of your head to touch the ceiling will elongate the spine, expand the rib cage and give your lungs more room to breathe. If you are in bed or lying down on the floor, the beach, or under a tree you can also follow some or all of the above suggestions.

Remember we are all human beings. We have all made mistakes, had regrets, and would have made different choices in our lives if we knew what we know now.

The most important action we can take right now is our next breath.

On that happy note, I wish you an interesting journey as you forge new trails up the mountains of life. I encourage you to share your trials and tribulations with your family, friends, and acquaintances so that we may all learn from your wisdom and experience. May we all take a deep breath, connect with our hearts, and reach out to the next being that crosses our path.

Namaste

Food for Thought

Teach us love, compassion, and honor,

that we may heal the earth and each other.

— Ojibwe Prayer

APPENDIX

Rx: Easy Does It – Mini-Movements

All of these suggestions may be done while standing, sitting, or lying down. Feel free to mix and match. There is no sacred order here.

1. Wiggle your toes towards face. Extra credit for pointing and flexing your feet!

2. Inhale as you squeeze your thighs, pause, exhale and release your thigh muscles.

3. Inhale, pull your belly button towards your spine, pause, exhale and release.

4. Inhale as you lift your shoulders up to your ears, pause and squeeze, then slowly exhale as you let your shoulders relax.

5. Inhale as you lift your chin up to the sky, pause, and then slowly bring your chin towards your chest. Pause as you pull shoulders down away from your ears. Then exhale and let your chin find a comfortable position.

6. Relax your jaw, open your mouth into a pretend yawn, and then let your face soften.

7. Inhale as you lift your toes towards your face, pause as you spread them as wide as they will go. Then slowly exhale, placing your toes gently back on the floor. If you are lying down, just let them go back to a relaxed position.

Rx: Questions to Ask Yourself Throughout the Day

1. Am I breathing?

2. What is the best use of my time right now?

3. What would I do right now if I knew I was going to die tonight?

4. Is there someone who I've been thinking about? Can I phone them? Send them a text, a note, or an email?

5. Is there something in my physical living space that I can give away today?

6. Are there dishes in the sink? Laundry to be done? Bills to be paid? Is there trash to be taken out to the garbage container or placed in the recycling bins?

7. Is this a good time to just sit for five minutes, focus on my breathing and recharge my batteries? This includes sitting silently or listening to music, observing a cat or dog sleeping, or watching a bird out the window.

Rx: 10 Quick Energy Infusions

1. **Stress Releases.** Inhale as you squeeze your hands into tight fists. Pause. Then slowly exhale and open your hands. Stretch your fingers as wide as possible. Feel free to repeat a few times.

2. **Sitting Kills.** The best antidote for sitting too long is to get up and move around. Stand up. Stretch. Jump up and down. Wiggle. Dance. Even if only for a few seconds. Make it a new habit.

3. **Lion's Pose.** Inhale, pause, and as you exhale, stick your tongue out as far as it will go. This is a wonderful stress releaser and if you want privacy, do it in the bathroom, your car, or when no one is looking. Three times is an absolute charm!

4. **Bathroom Mirror.** Make funny faces, stick your tongue out, wiggle, shake, get outrageous – it's just you and the mirror. Extra credit for smiling and laughing.

5. **Walking Tall.** Whenever you are walking outside or inside, see if you can roll your shoulders back and down, away from your ears. Feel your rib cage rise as you push the sky up with the top of your head.

6. **The Pause That Refreshes** (also known as taking a cigarette-less break!). Go outside or open a window. Take several deep breaths, remembering to concentrate on the pause between your inhales and your exhales.

7. **The power of ONE.** Do just one thing or one task at a time. This includes looking away from your computer screen, book, or newspaper as you take a sip of coffee or tea. Better yet, just sit and focus on that cup of tea or coffee, then go back to your current task.

8. **Giving.** Do something thoughtful for someone else. This includes making a phone call, sending a thoughtful email, or writing a handwritten note to someone you've been thinking about.

9. **Do absolutely NOTHING.** See if you can do this for one minute and maybe work up to three minutes. This is like an instant shower and you will be rewarded with an insight, or maybe a flash on where you put that piece of paper! My favorite is just lying on a carpeted floor on my back. If you have any back issues, just bend your knees or place a big pillow under them. If you need an assistant, find a cat or dog to be your practice buddy!

10. **SMILE.** This is an amazing technique, it works with friends, family, coworkers, strangers in the supermarket, and even on the telephone!

Rx: Mini-Meditation

Read through this section first, then come back and follow the instructions below.

1. **Find a comfortable seated position.** Close your eyes. You may want to take your glasses off and put them in a safe place. If closing your eyes is uncomfortable, you may want to experiment with keeping your eyes slightly closed, but if you do keep your eyes open make sure that they are soft and relaxed.

2. **Take a deep breath.** *Inhale, pause, exhale, and pause.* Continue breathing deeply and listen very closely. Can you acknowledge the static in your mind, let it go, and just focus on your inhales and exhales? For most of us this is very difficult. Who has time to stop, look, and listen when we have an endless list of errands, laundry, emails, housekeeping, dishes in the sink, bills to pay, work, shopping, yard work, and _____. (Fill in the blank. I am sure there is something on your list that popped right to the front of the line!)

3. **Tell whatever task,** item, or person that popped into your mind that you will get back to it in a few minutes. (If you are nervous you will forget, just jot yourself a quick note.)

4. **Picture in your mind** a person, place, or thing that really makes you happy. *A family member? A grandchild? A friend? The beach? A favorite trail?*

Summer camp as a kid? Skiing? Dancing? The tulips on the kitchen counter? A big bowl of ice cream? Reading a good book curled up by the fireplace? Your cat sunbathing in the window?

Hold that picture in your mind and just sit quietly breathing in and out as gently as you can. Do not worry about holding, pausing, or the lengths of your breaths. Just focus on your inhales and exhales. Take your time; this is all about just savoring your breath. Do not worry about the image or picture in your mind. It may fade, disappear, change, or morph into another image. It is just an anchor to get you started on experiencing your body breathing.

Continue gently breathing. Just savor what is happening and if your mind wanders, simply come back to your breath. See if you can just sit and breathe for a minute or two. You are most welcome to stay here as long as you choose. Just remember to focus on your happy image(s) and listen to your inhales and exhales.

When you are ready, open your eyes as slowly as possible and take a few more breaths to just enjoy the simple act of breathing.

Congratulations, you have just meditated!

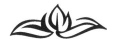

Rx: Plan a Lovely Meal with Friends

Plan a lovely meal with friends or family. Potlucks are my personal favorite because I don't feel pressured to invent a spectacular menu that will incorporate everyone's dietary preferences. Most people can handle making or purchasing one dish or contributing wine, cheese, bread, or dessert. Let people know you are working on enjoying a delicious, un-hurried and pleasant meal. Challenge the group to eat slowly and to spend more than an one hour eating together.

It also helps to set up boundaries, speak up if you get in-digestion with mixing politics, religion, or other issues with eating. One of the best dinner parties I ever hosted was one where we all recalled happy childhood moments. We all had an enjoyable time and learned more about each other. No one, including me, suffered indigestion or heartburn. The bottom line? Eat, chew, and listen!

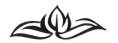

Yoga Rx: Chair Yoga

- When stretching, always remember it's an *inhale* as you lift your arms or legs up, and an *exhale* as you release back down to a neutral position.

- If you experience any sharp pains, please back off. Work with the body you have today.

- Please check in with a health care practitioner if you experience any discomfort or pain while doing any of these stretches.

- Remember that the slower you move in and out of these postures, the greater the relaxation benefit.

- Have fun and remember the following stretches are just suggestions; feel free to mix and match. If you find one routine that you really like, do it. There is no one-size-fits-all in breathing yoga postures.

1. **Release Eye Fatigue**

2. **Neck and Shoulder Stretches**

3. **Hand and Wrist Stretches**

4. **Releasing Jaw Tension**

5. **Feet and Ankle Stretches**

6. **Lower Back Stretches**

1. Release Eye Fatigue

1. **Soften your eyes.** Rotate both eyes up to the ceiling, to the far right, down towards the floor, to the far left, and back to the ceiling. Then do the opposite rotation, far left, down to the floor, far right, and back towards the ceiling. Gently close your eyes and enjoy letting your eyes taking a much-needed rest.

2. **Refocus.** Inhale and squeeze both eyes tightly. Notice that your face may naturally squinch up into a prune or raisin face. Pause. And then exhale and release your face and let your eyes soften. Let your shoulders relax.

3. **Breathing is easier when you let your face relax.** You will notice that smiling not only relaxes the body, but also makes it easier to breathe.

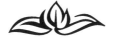

2. Neck and Shoulder Stretches

1. **Ear to shoulder.** Inhale, pause, and then exhale, dropping your right ear towards your right shoulder. Pause and enjoy the stretch on your left side of your neck. On your next inhale let your head float back up to center, pause, and slowly drop your ear towards your left shoulder. Feel free to do this several times as you release neck and should tensions.

2. **Chin to collarbone.** After a deep inhale, pause, and then as you exhale, slowly drop your chin to your chest. Feel free to relax into this posture using your inhales, pauses, and exhales to release any tension in the back of the neck, shoulders, and upper back. When you are ready to release, inhale and slowly lift your chin back to its normal resting place.

3. **Hands behind the head.** Interlace your fingers and place them on the back of your head. Slowly move your elbows to push behind you as you feel your chest lift, open, and expand. If it is safe to do so, you may want to lean back a little bit and enjoy the sensation of opening the chest. If you have had recent shoulder or heart surgery, be sure to clear this one with your health care provider.

3. *Hand and Wrist Stretches*

NOTE: *These stretches are great to do if you have been using your hands and need to give them a break from writing, gardening, chopping vegetables, woodworking, knitting, etc.*

- **Prayer Position I.** Inhale as you press your palms together, pause, exhale and release. You can do this a few times without actually separating your hands. This is a great tension releaser and it will also strengthen your forearm muscles without lifting weights.

- **Prayer Position II.** Pressing your palms together, gently bend your fingers to the right and then to the left. Extra credit for using your inhales and exhales as you move from right, to center, and then to left. This one can also be done in public, especially while sitting in a meeting, church, or waiting for an appointment. This is definitely an instant stress releaser!

- **Fists to Flowers.** Inhale and squeeze your hands into a fist, pause, and then as you exhale, stretch your fingers as widely as they will go today. Sometimes I like to stretch my arms out to the side as I make fists and then release all ten fingers. Listen to your body, it may choose some movement you may have not even imagined!

- **Interlace Fingers.** Stretch your arms out in front of you, overhead (if you are injury free), and then gently sway your arms side-to-side. Be sure to keep breathing!

- **Hula Hands.** Move your arms, hands, and fingers as if you were doing a hula. This can be done sitting down – or if you choose to stand up, feel free to move your hips and feet! Extra credit for smiling!

4. Releasing Jaw Tension

- **Lion Pose.** Inhale, pause, and on an exhale stick your tongue out as far as it will go, pause, and then inhale back to neutral. Feel free to add a roar or a growl! When I am having a rough day, I do several lion poses in the bathroom in front of a mirror and usually wind up laughing because it releases so much tension.

- **Pretend** you are chewing gum!

- **Wear a soft smile** as you go about your day and notice how you feel. Smile like you have the secret to the universe… and you do – it's in your smile.

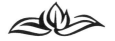

5. Feet and Ankle Stretches

NOTE: *If you have had foot or ankle surgery, please check with your health care practitioner before doing the following stretches.*

- **Point/Flex Feet.** This stretch is great to do when seated in cars, theaters, airplanes, and meetings. Simply point your toes away from you and then point your toes toward your face.

- **Ankle Rotations.** If possible, kick your shoes off and make circle rotations with your left ankle, and then your right ankle. Be sure to circle to the right and then to the left. Notice that one side may be easier than the other. You can even add more fun by trying to rotate both ankles at the same time!

- **Ballet.** Inhale as you rise up on your toes, pause, then exhale slowly as you lower your heels back to the floor. This one is great to do holding onto a bathroom or kitchen sink, or the back of a chair for support.

6. Lower Back Stretches

NOTE: *If you have had any back injuries or surgeries, please check with your health care practitioner before doing the following stretches.*

- **Bend Forward.** Sitting on your chair, inhale as you lift your chest, pause, and then slowly exhale your chest towards your thighs. Sometimes it feels better to separate the knees. Don't worry about how far you can go. You can place your hands on the side of the chair for added stability. This is about giving the spine a chance to release. If you can lower your chest to your thighs, then place your hands on the floor and gently shake out your head. Remember to use your inhales and exhales as you slowly return to a seated position.

- **Ankle to Opposite Knee.** Seated on a firm chair, inhale and place your right ankle so that it is resting on your left knee. Pause and continue to mindfully breathe. When you are ready to switch sides, simply inhale as you lift your ankle, and exhale as you place your foot back on the floor. Be sure to do both sides. This is a good time to point and flex your feet or give them a mini massage.

- **Practice Sitting Straight.** Sit up straight and tall on the edge of a firm chair, continue breathing as you pull your shoulders down and away from your ears, then gently lift the crown of your head towards the sky.

Rx: Unfinished Business

NOTE: *These are just suggestions. This list is NOT in order of importance.*

- Have I shared the following three feelings with all the people in my life that I need to:

  1) *Thank you.*

  2) *I love you.*

  3) *I am sorry.*

- Are my finances in order? Are my debts paid off? Do I have a plan in place for handling my finances when I am no longer capable, am incapacitated, or have died?

- Do my loved ones know my final wishes, including end-of-life decisions, funeral plans, and where to find my Last Will & Testament? Please make sure everything is written down so that your family, friends, physicians, and attorneys have accurate information. On an annual basis remind the appropriate people of this info and let them know if you have made any changes in your documents.

- Have I given away all the material things that I do not need, love, or want at this time in my life? Remember if you live with other beings, please respect their need to keep their material possessions.

Rx: Angst

You just found out that you are going to die tomorrow morning. What angst is left on your plate? Is there any issue, person, or incident that is still bothering you? How important is it that you resolve it?

What can you let go of and what can you change? Are you holding on to any lies of omission? Are you NOT telling the truth, when it would make a positive change for the better?

Please remember that you do NOT have to contact this person; indeed, they may be dead. But being honest with yourself may allow for some much-needed healing. This is often an uncomfortable place. However painful, the truth will set you free.

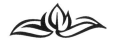

Rx: The Conversation –
End-of-Life Topics

Please note that I am not a bioethicist; however, I firmly believe that discussing your end-of-life preferences on your death bed may not be the best place to start this conversation.

You will find a wealth of information on this topic in the library, in bookstores, and on the internet. Some of it is misleading, but I trust that you are a wise individual who will choose what is best for you. Be sure to revisit this conversation on a regular basis with your loved ones.

The media offer daily news, often with heart-wrenching and heartfelt stories that offer a natural base for discussing end-of-life issues with your friends and family. You may also have your own story about someone who did not make their wishes known and suffered needlessly.

Important topics for discussion include:

- Organ and tissue donation.
- Not starting treatment and/or stopping treatment.
- Artificial hydration and nutrition.
- Hospice care.
- Palliative/comfort care.
- Voluntary stop eating and drinking (VSED).
- Palliative sedation.
- POLST (Physician orders for life-sustaining treatment).
- Body disposition: green burial, burial or cremation, including disposition of cremains.

If you are having difficulty starting this conversation, begin by asking yourself, your loved ones, and friends: "*Is being brain dead the same as being dead?*" Review the cases of Karen Ann Quinlan, Terri Schiavo, Bobbi Kristina Brown, and Jahi McMath. You may even have some people you know personally or have heard of in your circle of friends, family, or acquaintances.

It is your responsibility to start the conversation. Please remember that some of your friends and family may be horrified, angry, or upset with you. It is important to love, trust and honor them, hoping they can at least listen to your final requests, even if they disagree with you.

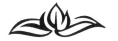

Rx: Checklist for Organizing Your Personal Information

NOTE: *There are many resources available, including books, binders, and online organizers that can help you collect your documents. You may also choose to use a notebook, thumb drive, DVD, or the Cloud to store your information. Remember that storage technology changes and your choice of storage needs to be current.*

Whatever methodology you use, just make sure that at least two trusted people know how to retrieve the information. If it's not ALL in one place, be sure to list where the documents can be found. Do not use your cell phone to store all this data unless it is backed up to the Cloud and your designated people can access it. Also, cell phones can break, get lost, or stolen.

The list may be daunting, and so I highly recommend doing one task a day or weekly. Please remember that this is just an outline. Some items are listed twice, under different categories, simply because we all have different filing systems. Remember that EVERY situation is unique, so feel free to modify this list in any way that works for you. **One of the most valuable legacies you can leave your loved ones is to have your house in order BEFORE you die.** And please do not forget to include what happens to your pets if you are hospitalized, incapacitated, or die.

Personal Records

- **Full Legal Name.** Include your maiden name and/or past legal names.

- **Date of Birth.** Copy of your birth certificate, with the original in a safe place.

- **Birthplace.** Also include names of parents and siblings.

- **Social Security Number.**

- **Legal Residence.** (If you live in multiple places, be sure to list all relevant information.)

- **Contact Information.** Names, addresses, phone numbers, and email addresses. (List of spouse/ significant other, children, siblings, relatives, best friends, and whoever you would like to be contacted in case of an accident, serious illness, or death.)

- **Location of Documents.** Birth, marriage, divorce, citizenship, adoption, passport, social security card, bank accounts, stocks/bonds, retirement funds, property deeds, property taxes, etc.

- **Employers.** If you are retired you may want to list only a few employers or occupations.

- **Education.**

- **Military Records.**

- **Memberships.** Organizations including active affiliations in church, volunteer activities, social, political, and environmental groups, including awards.

- **Professional Contacts.** Full name, address, phone numbers, and email: accountant, attorney, financial advisors, health care providers, including your primary physician and other specialists.

- **Medications.** Be sure to carry a list in your wallet/cell phone and update the list whenever your medications and/or dosages change. Most pharmacies will give you a printout of your current prescriptions. Be sure to list the name of pharmacy/pharmacies and list any medications that you are receiving via mail order; include contact numbers and medication names so that these can be adjusted or canceled.

- **Location of Important Items.** Home/office safe, safety deposit box and key, home/car/office keys, and security codes.

- **Financial Records.** Be sure to update the beneficiary status on all your accounts. Let your financial institutions know who will be contacting them if you are dealing with a serious illness or have died. Your Durable Power of Attorney will have the necessary documentation. If you are in a small community, and/or have a personal relationship with any of your financial institutions, it is a courtesy to let them know that you have updated your records.

- **Income.** Employer, retirement accounts, IRAs, 401(k), trusts, etc. Use your current statements from all your financial institutions for easy reference.

- **Medicare/Medicaid/Dental** Insurance cards, including all current health insurance documents.

- **Bank accounts.** Names of all financial institutions and account numbers.

- **Investments.** Stocks, bonds, property, and certificates: location, account information, and contact information including stockbrokers' names.

- **Income Tax.** Most recent income tax return; this will offer a glimpse of your financial portrait. Be sure to update your files yearly so that it will be easier for your after-death team.

- **Last Will and Testament,** including Durable Power of Attorney.

- **Life and Accident Insurance Plans.** Policy paperwork.

- **Medical Directives.** Durable Power of Attorney for Healthcare, End of Life Advance Directive, POLST (Physician's Orders for Life Sustaining Treatment), and for Alzheimer's Disease – Dementia Mental Health Advance Directive.

- **Home(s).** Location of original loan(s), deeds, including any property tax documentation.

- **Transportation.** Location of titles and registration for vehicles, boats, motorcycles, airplanes, including outstanding loans. Bonus points for including insurance and maintenance records so that your after-death team will have an easier time donating or selling your assets.

- **Credit/Debit Cards.** Account numbers, addresses, and any access codes, so that any balances can be paid.

- **Funeral/Obituary.** Preferred mortuary or burial society, including name of cemetery, green burial site, or cremation. If you don't care where you are buried or your ashes are scattered, be sure to put that in writing, preferably signed and dated. If you want a gravestone, be sure to include your epitaph. Even if you choose not to put an obituary in the newspaper or on your social media account, it is helpful to your loved ones if you write it before you die. I have written two obituaries, one for the public and one for friends and family. This may seem depressing; however, I see it as life affirming, a wake-up call-to-action with whatever time we have left!

Miscellaneous (and just as important)

- **Pet care.** Leave a detailed plan for the care of your pets. Include feeding instructions, medications, veterinarian, and any other information that will help the caregiver. If possible, see if you can find friends and family who agree to adopt your pet(s) in the event that you are hospitalized, incapacitated, or die.

- **Cyberspace.** Location of computer logins and passwords, including all your social media accounts.

FINAL NOTE: *As you go through this list, you may think of more items. The most important thing is to start right now. I guarantee you will feel better, lighter, and freer once you have all of the above in one place for your loved ones to access when the time comes.*

Rx: Understanding Grief – The Index Card Exercise

WARNING: *This is a very powerful exercise. Feel free to stop at any time and notice your feelings, emotions, and insights. This exercise is designed to make us more aware and sensitive to all that we love and all that we care about. What you do with the answers is totally up to you.*

1. Find a quiet place where you will not be interrupted.

2. Place an empty bowl, tray, plate, or basket in front of you.

3. Take ten index cards or small pieces of paper and write down the top ten people, places, or activities that you absolutely love.

4. Remember that nothing is set in stone, this is just an exercise.

5. Lay out all the cards in front of you.

6. Choose one card that you could live without and place it in the empty container.

7. Take a deep breath and choose another card that you could live without.

8. Continue until you get through nine cards and then **STOP**.

9. Notice that you are holding onto card number ten. Be aware of your feelings, emotions, and most likely tears.

10. Slowly place the last card in the container and close your eyes.

11. Take your time and notice what comes up for you.

12. Be open to the answer within.

13. I personally like to transition back into my everyday life with a journal entry, a bath/shower, or a walk. Whatever you do, do it mindfully, with love and attention.

Food for Thought

When I was young and free and my imagination had

no limits, I dreamed of changing the world.

As I grew older and wiser, I discovered the world would

not change, so I shortened my sights somewhat and

decided to change only my country.

But it, too, seemed immovable.

As I grew into my twilight years, in one last desperate

attempt, I settled for changing only my family, those

closest to me, but alas, they would have none of it.

And now, as I lie on my deathbed, I suddenly realize:

If I had only changed myself first,

then by example I would have changed my family.

From their inspiration and encouragement, I would

then have been able to better my country, and who

knows, I may have even changed the world.

— Epitaph on the tomb of an Anglican Bishop
in Westminster Abbey (1100 A.D.)

About the Author

MARGARET CHESTER, MPH, RYT, has more than 50 years practicing yoga with a working background in the health care field. She has created a versatile yoga practice for ageless seniors that fosters ease, vitality and a zest for living on and off the mat. As Margaret likes to say: "If you can breathe, you can do this yoga!"

Other Books by The Author

Chocolate Yoga: A System of Yoga Techniques for Stress and Weight Management That Will Nurture Your Body, Mind and Spirit.

Are you stressed, tired, unhappy and feeling out of control? **Chocolate Yoga** is a system of yoga techniques that anyone can use to address stress and weight issues to nurture your body, mind, and spirit.

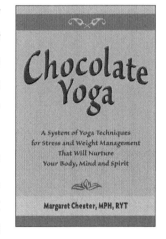

The idea of **Chocolate Yoga** is to be able to live more in the moment. **Chocolate Yoga** is a feeling. It can best be described as a sense of peace. It is that first bite of chocolate. It is that sensation that just melts in your mouth and travels through your body. Of course it usually feels so good we want more.

The basic postures and breathing exercises are easy to do whether you have three minutes or thirty minutes. No special equipment or mats are needed. This program is highly recommended to anyone who has tried yoga and found it hard, complicated, or intimidating.

If you are experiencing low energy, depression, or fatigue, this yoga will energize and motivate you. **Chocolate Yoga** will give you increased flexibility, balance, focus, strength, and relaxation as you practice these techniques throughout your busy day.

This program is based on the idea that stress and weight issues are flip sides of the same coin. If you manage your stress you will be able to manage your weight issues. *Chocolate Yoga* will give you a lifetime of pleasure, health, and happiness.

The Chocolate Yoga Action Workbook.

This action workbook is based on the five principles of *Chocolate Yoga.* We all know that life is often not easy, fair, or fun. It is often messy, confusing, and upsetting. Yet most of us are yearning for more peace, happiness, and freedom in our everyday lives. And your answers are waiting within.

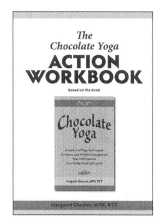

Why a workbook? Because life is work. And you **are** your life's work. No one else is going to do your inner work. Here are some tools and exercises to help you find more peace and serenity in your everyday life.

It all starts with asking yourself: *Where am I right now? Where do I want to go? How am I going to get there?* You will find your answers as you dig into the action exercises in this workbook. Each exercise is designed to take your body, mind and spirit to the next level.

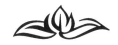

For More Information:
www.ChocolateYoga.com

53264473R00087

Made in the USA
Columbia, SC
13 March 2019